UNDERGROUND
CLINICAL VIGNETTES

······································

MICROBIOLOGY VOL. II

Classic Clinical Cases for
USMLE Step 1 Review [105 cases, 1st ed]

VIKAS BHUSHAN, MD
University of California, San Francisco, Class of 1991
Series Editor, Diagnostic Radiologist

CHIRAG AMIN, MD
University of Miami, Class of 1996
Orlando Regional Medical Center, Resident in Orthopaedic Surgery

TAO LE, MD
University of California, San Francisco, Class of 1996
Yale-New Haven Hospital, Resident in Internal Medicine

HOANG NGUYEN
Northwestern University, Class of 2000

VISHAL PALL, MBBS
Government Medical College, Chandigarh, India, Class of 1996

SONAL SHAH
Ross University, Class of 2000

DISTRIBUTED by Blackwell Science
Editorial Offices:
350 Main Street, Malden, Massachusetts 02148, USA

DISTRIBUTORS

USA

Blackwell Science, Inc.
Commerce Place
350 Main Street
Malden, Massachusetts 02148
Telephone orders: (+1 877-727-7722)

Australia

Blackwell Science Pty., Ltd.
54 University Street
Carlton, Victoria 3053

Canada

Login Brothers Book Company
324 Saulteaux Crescent
Winnipeg, Manitoba
Canada, R3J 3T2

Outside North America and Australia

Blackwell Science, Ltd.
c/o Marston Book Services, Ltd.
P.O. Box 269, Abingdon
Oxon, OX14 4YN England

EDITOR: Andrea Fellows

TYPESETTER: Vikas Bhushan using MS Word97

© 1999 by S2S Medical Publishing
Printed and bound by Capital City Press
Printed in the United States of America

ISBN: 1-890061-30-1

Contributors

....

RICHA VARMA
Cambridge University, Class of 2001

ASHRAF ZAMAN, MBBS
New Delhi, India

VIPAL SONI
UCLA School of Medicine, Class of 1999

Faculty Reviewer

....

WARREN LEVINSON, MD, PHD
Professor of Microbiology and Immunology, UCSF School of Medicine

Acknowledgments

. . . .

Throughout the production of this book, we have had the support of many friends and colleagues. Special thanks to our business manager, Gianni Le Nguyen. For expert computer support, Tarun Mathur and Alex Grimm. For design suggestions, Sonia Santos and Elizabeth Sanders.

For editing, proofreading, and assistance across the vignette series, we collectively thank Carolyn Alexander, Henry E. Aryan, Natalie Barteneva, Sanjay Bindra, Julianne Brown, Hebert Chen, Arnold Chin, Yoon Cho, Karekin R. Cunningham, A. Sean Dalley, Sunit Das, Ryan Armando Dave, Robert DeMello, David Donson, Alea Eusebio, Priscilla A. Frase, Anil Gehi, Parul Goyal, Alex Grimm, Tim Jackson, Sundar Jayaraman, Aarchan Joshi, Rajni K. Jutla, Faiyaz Kapadi, Aaron S. Kesselheim, Sana Khan, Andrew Pin-wei Ko, Warren S. Krackov, Benjamin H.S. Lau, Scott Lee, Warren Levinson, Eric Ley, Ken Lin, Samir Mehta, Gil Melmed, Joe Messina, Vivek Nandkarni, Deanna Nobleza, Darin T. Okuda, Adam L. Palance, Sonny Patel, Ricardo Pietrobon, Riva L. Rahl, Aashita Randeria, Marilou Reyes, Diego Ruiz, Anthony Russell, Sanjay Sahgal, Sonal Shah, John Stulak, Lillian Su, Julie Sundaram, Rita Suri, Richa Varma, Amy Williams, Ashraf Zaman and David Zipf. Please let us know if your name has been missed or mispelled and we will be happy to make the change in the next edition.

Table of Contents

. . . .

CASE	SUBSPECIALTY	NAME
40	ID	Chlamydia Pneumonia
41	ID	Colorado Tick Fever
42	ID	Crimean-Congo Hemorrhagic Fever
43	ID	Croup
44	ID	Dengue Hemorrhagic Fever
45	ID	Ebola Virus Hemorrhagic Fever
46	ID	Ehrlichiosis
47	ID	Endemic Typhus
48	ID	Gonococcal Ophthalmia Neonatorum
49	ID	Gram-Negative Sepsis
50	ID	Granuloma Inguinale
51	ID	*H. influenzae* in a COPD Patient
52	ID	Hantavirus Pulmonary Syndrome
53	ID	Hemorrhagic Fever Renal Syndrome
54	ID	Herpangina
55	ID	Herpes Zoster Ophthalmicus
56	ID	HSV Keratitis
57	ID	Inclusion Conjunctivitis
58	ID	Influenza
59	ID	Jarisch–Herxheimer Reaction
60	ID	Kawasaki Syndrome
61	ID	Lepromatous Leprosy
62	ID	Leptospirosis (Weil's Disease)
63	ID	Miliary Tuberculosis
64	ID	Necrotizing Fasciitis
65	ID	Nosocomial Enterococcal Infection
66	ID	Otitis Externa
67	ID	Overwhelming Postsplenectomy Infections
68	ID	Proctocolitis
69	ID	Psittacosis
70	ID	Q Fever
71	ID	Rat Bite Fever
72	ID	Relapsing Fever
73	ID	RSV Pneumonia
74	ID	*Salmonella* Septicemia with Osteomyelitis
75	ID	Scabies
76	ID	Tetanus Neonatorum
77	ID	Tick Paralysis
78	ID	Trachoma
79	ID	Traumatic Gas Gangrene
80	ID	Yaws
81	Neurology	Amebic Meningoencephalitis
82	Neurology	Brain Abscess with Heart Disease
83	Neurology	Herpes Simplex Encephalitis
84	Neurology	Japanese Encephalitis
85	Neurology	*Listeria* Meningitis in the Newborn
86	Neurology	Lymphocytic Choriomeningitis (LCM)
87	Neurology	Progressive Multifocal

CASE	SUBSPECIALTY	NAME
88	Neurology	Ramsay Hunt Syndrome
89	Neurology	Reye's Syndrome
90	Neurology	St. Louis Encephalitis
91	Neurology	Subacute Sclerosing Panencephalitis
92	Neurology	Tubercular Meningitis
93	OB/Gyn	Bacterial Vaginosis
94	OB/Gyn	Breast Abscess
95	OB/Gyn	Chorioamnionitis
96	OB/Gyn	HIV Transmission in Pregnancy
97	OB/Gyn	Pelvic Inflammatory Disease (PID)
98	OB/Gyn	Toxic Shock Syndrome (TSS)
99	OB/Gyn	Tubercular Salpingitis
100	Urology	Acute Prostatitis
101	Urology	Chronic Prostatitis
102	Urology	Epididymitis
103	Urology	Poststreptococcal Glomerulonephritis
104	Urology	Urinary Schistosomiasis
105	Urology	UTI with *Staphylococcus saprophyticus*

Preface

. . . .

This series was developed to address the increasing number of clinical vignette questions on the USMLE Step 1. It is designed to supplement and complement *First Aid for the USMLE Step 1* (Appleton & Lange). Bi-directional cross-linking to appropriate High Yield Facts in the 1999 edition has been implemented

Each book uses a series of approximately 100 "**supra-prototypical**" **cases as a way to condense testable facts and associations.** The clinical vignettes in this series are designed to incorporate as many testable facts as possible into a cohesive and memorable clinical picture. The vignettes represent composites drawn from general and specialty textbooks, reference books, thousands of USMLE style questions and the personal experience of the authors and reviewers.

Although each case tends to present all the signs, symptoms, and diagnostic findings for a particular illness, **patients generally will not present with such a "complete" picture either clinically or on the Step 1 exam**. Cases are not meant to simulate a potential real patient or an exam vignette. All the **boldfaced "buzzwords" are for learning purposes** and are not necessarily expected to be found in any one patient with the disease.

Definitions of selected important terms are placed within the vignettes in (= SMALL CAPS) in parentheses. Other parenthetical remarks often refer to the pathophysiology or mechanism of disease. The format should also help students learn to present cases succinctly during oral "bullet" presentations on clinical rotations. The cases are meant to be read as a condensed review, not as a primary reference.

The information provided in this book has been prepared with a great deal of thought and careful research. This book should not, however, be considered as your sole source of information.

We invite your corrections and suggestions for the next edition of this book. For the first submission of each factual correction or new vignette, you will receive a personal acknowledgement and a free copy of the revised book. We prefer that you submit corrections or suggestions via electronic mail to vbhushan@aol.com. Please include "Underground Vignettes" as the subject of your message. If you do not have access to e-mail, use the following mailing address: S2S Medical Publishing, 1015 Gayley Ave, Box 1113, Los Angeles, CA 90024 USA.

Abbreviations

. . . .

ABGs – arterial blood gases
ABPA – allergic bronchopulmonary aspergillosis
ADA – adenosine deaminase
AIDS – acquired immunodeficiency syndrome
ALT – alanine transaminase
Angio – angiography
ARC – AIDS-related complex
ARDS – acute respiratory distress syndrome
ASO – antistreptolysin O
AST – aspartate transaminase
AZT - zidovudine
BCG – bacille Calmette-Guérin
BE – barium enema
BP – blood pressure
BUN – blood urea nitrogen
cAMP – cyclic adenosine monophosphate
CBC – complete blood count
cGMP – cyclic guanosine monophosphate
CLL – chronic lymphocytic leukemia
CMV - cytomegalovirus
CSF – cerebrospinal fluid
CT – computerized tomography
CXR – chest x-ray
DIC – disseminated intravascular coagulation
DTRs – deep tendon reflexes
ECG – electrocardiography
Echo - echocardiography
EEG – electroencephalography
EGD – esophagogastroduodenoscopy
EHEC – enterohemorrhagic *E. coli*
ELISA – enzyme-linked immunosorbent assay
EMG – electromyography
EPVE – early prosthetic valve endocarditis
ERCP – endoscopic retrograde cholangiopancreatography
ESR – erythrocyte sedimentation rate
ETEC – enterotoxigenic *E. coli*
FNA – fine needle aspiration
FTA-ABS – fluorescent treponemal antibody absorption
GVHD – graft-versus-host disease
Hb - hemoglobin
HFMD – hand, foot, and mouth disease
HIDA – hepato-iminodiacetic acid [scan]
HIV – human immunodeficiency virus
HPF – high-power field
HPI – history of present illness
HSG – hysterosalpingography
HSV – herpes simplex virus
ID/CC – identification and chief complaint
Ig - immunoglobulin

Abbreviations - continued

IVP – intravenous pyelography
KOH – potassium hydroxide
KUB – kidneys/ureter/bladder
LCM – lymphocytic choriomeningitis
LDH – lactate dehydrogenase
LMN – lower motor neuron
LP – lumbar puncture
LPVE – late prosthetic valve endocarditis
LT – labile toxin
Lytes – electrolytes
Mammo – mammography
MR – magnetic resonance [imaging]
Nuc – nuclear medicine
PA – posteroanterior
PBS – peripheral blood smear
PCR – polymerase chain reaction
PE – physical exam
PET – positron emission tomography
PFTs – pulmonary function tests
PID – pelvic inflammatory disease
PMC – pseudomembranous colitis
PMN - polymorphonuclear leukocyte
PT – prothrombin time
PTT – partial thromboplastin time
RBC – red blood cell
RPR – rapid plasma reagin
RR – respiratory rate
SBFT – small bowel follow-through [barium study]
SCID – severe combined immunodeficiency
SSPE – subacute sclerosing panencephalitis
ST – stable toxin
STD – sexually transmitted disease
TSS – toxic shock syndrome
TSST – toxic shock syndrome toxin
UA – urinalysis
UGI – upper GI [barium study]
US – ultrasound
UTI – urinary tract infection
V/Q – ventilation perfusion
VDRL – Venereal Disease Research Laboratory
VS – vital signs
VSD – ventricular septal defect
WBC – white blood cell
XR – x-ray

ID/CC	A 25-year-old **IV drug abuser** presents with a **high fever** with chills, malaise, a productive cough, hemoptysis, and right-sided pleuritic chest pain.
HPI	He also reports multiple skin infections at injection sites.
PE	VS: fever. PE: **stigmata of intravenous drug abuse** at multiple injection sites; skin infections; thrombosed peripheral veins; **splenomegaly and pulsatile hepatomegaly; ejection systolic murmur,** increasing with inspiration, heard in tricuspid area.
Labs	CBC: normochromic, normocytic anemia. UA: microscopic hematuria. Blood culture yields *S. aureus.*
Imaging	Echo: presence of **vegetations on tricuspid valve** and **tricuspid incompetence.** CXR: consolidation.
Gross Pathology	N/A
Micro Pathology	N/A
Treatment	**High-dose intravenous penicillinase-resistant penicillin** in combination with an **aminoglycoside.** If isolated, *S. aureus* strain is **methicillin resistant,** and **vancomycin** is the drug of choice.
Discussion	In drug addicts, the tricuspid valve is the site of infection more frequently (55%) than the aortic valve (35%) or the mitral valve (30%); these findings contrast markedly with the rarity of right-sided involvement in cases of infective endocarditis that are not associated with drug abuse. *S. aureus* is responsible for the majority of cases. Certain organisms have a predilection for particular valves in cases of addict-associated endocarditis; for example, enterococci, other streptococcal species, and non-albicans *Candida* organisms predominantly affect the valves of the left side of the heart, while *S. aureus* infects valves on both the right and the left side of the heart. *Pseudomonas* organisms are associated with biventricular and multiple valve infection in addicts.

ID/CC	A 64-year-old male presents with rapidly **progressive dyspnea and fever.**
HPI	He has a history of orthopnea and paroxysmal nocturnal dyspnea and also reports pink, frothy sputum (= HEMOPTYSIS). One month ago he underwent a **bioprosthetic valve replacement** for calcific aortic stenosis. He is not hypertensive and has never had overt cardiac failure in the past.
PE	VS: fever; hypotension. PE: bilateral basal inspiratory crepts heard; cardiac auscultation suggestive of **aortic incompetence** (early diastolic murmur heard radiating down left sternal edge).
Labs	Three consecutive blood cultures yield **coagulase-negative S. epidermidis;** strain found to be **methicillin resistant.**
Imaging	CXR (PA view): suggestive of **pulmonary edema.** Echo: confirms presence of **prosthetic aortic valve dehiscence** leading to incompetence and poor left ventricular function.
Gross Pathology	N/A
Micro Pathology	N/A
Treatment	High-dose parenteral antibiotics— vancomycin (drug of choice for methicillin-resistant *S. aureus*), gentamycin, and oral rifampicin; surgical replacement of damaged prosthetic valve
Discussion	Prosthetic valve endocarditis is subdivided into two categories: early prosthetic valve endocarditis (EPVE), which becomes clinically manifest within 60 days after valve replacement (most commonly caused by *S. epidermidis,* followed by gram-negative bacilli and *Candida*), and late prosthetic valve endocarditis (LPVE), which is manifested clinically > 60 days after valve replacement (most commonly caused by viridans *Streptococci*). **FIRST AID** p.182

PROSTHETIC VALVE ENDOCARDITIS

ID/CC	A 54-year-old female who **underwent** a left mastectomy with **axillary lymph node dissection** a year ago presents with **pain** together with rapidly spreading **redness** and **swelling** of the left **arm**.
HPI	One year ago, she was diagnosed and operated on for stage 1 **carcinoma of the left breast**.
PE	Left forearm swollen, indurated, pink, and markedly tender; overlying temperature raised; margins and borders of skin lesion ill defined and not elevated (vs. erysipelas).
Labs	Needle aspiration from advancing border of the lesion, when stained and cultured, isolated **beta-hemolytic group A** streptococcus.
Imaging	N/A
Gross Pathology	N/A
Micro Pathology	N/A
Treatment	Penicillin.
Discussion	Cellulitis is an acute spreading infection of the skin that predominantly affects deeper subcutaneous tissue. **Group A streptococci and** *S. aureus* are the **most common** etiologic agents in adults; *H. influenzae* infection is common in children. Patients with chronic venous stasis and lymphedema of any cause (lymphoma, filariasis, post–regional lymph node dissection) are predisposed; recently, recurrent saphenous-vein donor-site cellulitis was found to be attributable to group A, C, or G streptococci.

. . . .

CELLULITIS

ID/CC	A 30-year-old **slaughterhouse worker** presents with a **painful, red swelling** of the **index finger** of his right hand.
HPI	The swelling developed four days after he was **injured** with a knife **while slaughtering a pig.**
PE	Well-defined, exquisitely tender, slightly elevated **violaceous lesion seen on right index finger;** no suppuration noted; right epitrochlear and right axillary lymphadenopathy noted.
Labs	Biopsy from edge of lesion yields *Erysipelothrix rhusiopathiae,* a thin, pleomorphic, nonsporulating, microaerophilic gram-positive rod.
Imaging	N/A
Gross Pathology	N/A
Micro Pathology	N/A
Treatment	**Penicillin G** or ciprofloxacin in penicillin-allergic patients.
Discussion	Erysipeloid refers to **localized cellulitis,** usually of the fingers and hands, caused by *Erysipelothrix rhusiopathiae;* infection in humans is usually the result of **contact with infected animals** or their products. Organisms gain entry via cuts and abrasions on the skin.

ERYSIPELOID

ID/CC	A **10-year-old** male complains of a spreading **skin rash** and **painful** swelling of both **wrists.**
HPI	The patient's mother states that the rash began with **erythema of the cheeks** (= "SLAPPED-CHEEK APPEARANCE") and subsequently progressed to involve the trunk and limbs.
PE	**Erythematous lacy/reticular skin rash** involving face, trunk, and limbs; bilateral swelling and painful restriction of movement at both **wrist joints.**
Labs	Serology detects presence of **specific IgM antibody to parvovirus;** ASO titer (to rule out acute rheumatic fever) normal; rheumatoid factor (to rule out rheumatoid arthritis) negative.
Imaging	N/A
Gross Pathology	N/A
Micro Pathology	N/A
Treatment	Self-limiting disease.
Discussion	A small (20- to 26-nm), **single-stranded DNA virus, parvovirus B19** causes erythema infectiosum (fifth disease) in schoolchildren, **aplastic crises** in persons with underlying hemolytic disorders (e.g., sickle cell anemia), **chronic anemia** in immunocompromised hosts, and **fetal loss** in pregnant women.

ID/CC	A 30-year-old male presents with a mildly pruritic **skin rash on the trunk, upper arm, and neck.**
HPI	The patient is otherwise in excellent health.
PE	Multiple **hypopigmented, scaling, confluent macules** seen on **trunk, upper arms, and neck;** no sensory loss demonstrated over areas of hypopigmentation; **Wood's lamp** examination of skin macules displays a **pale yellow to blue-white fluorescence.**
Labs	Examination of KOH mounting of scales from lesions demonstrates the presence of short, thick, tangled hyphae with clusters of large, spherical budding yeast cells with characteristic **"spaghetti-and-meatballs"** appearance.
Imaging	N/A
Gross Pathology	N/A
Micro Pathology	N/A
Treatment	**Topical selenium sulfide;** antifungal agents such as **miconazole** and **clotrimazole;** oral itraconazole in recalcitrant cases.
Discussion	Tinea versicolor, common in young adults, is a relatively asymptomatic superficial skin infection caused by the lipophilic organism *Pityrosporum orbiculare* (also termed *Malassezia furfur*). The lesions, which usually have a follicular origin, are small, hypopigmented-to-tan macules with a branlike furfuraceous scale; the macules are distributed predominantly on areas of the body predisposed to seborrhea, such as the **upper trunk, neck, shoulders, and face.**

PITYRIASIS VERSICOLOR

ID/CC   A 20-year-old male from **India** presents to the ER with **severe nausea and vomiting.**

HPI   Careful history reveals that two hours ago he ate some **unrefrigerated fried rice** that his wife had cooked the night before. He does not complain of any fever or diarrhea (may or may not be present).

PE   VS: no fever. PE: mild dehydration; diffuse mild abdominal tenderness.

Labs   Fecal staining reveals no RBCs, WBCs, or parasites; *Bacillus cereus,* **a gram-positive rod,** isolated from vomitus and stool and shown to produce the **emetogenic enterotoxin.**

Imaging   N/A

Gross Pathology   N/A

Micro Pathology   N/A

Treatment   Supportive.

Discussion   *Bacillus cereus* causes two distinct syndromes: a **diarrheal form** (mediated by an *E. coli* LT-type enterotoxin with an incubation period of 8–16 hours; caused by meats and vegetables) and an **emetic form** (mediated by an *S. aureus*-type enterotoxin with an incubation period of 1–8 hours; caused by fried rice). Proper food handling and refrigeration of boiled rice are largely preventive.

BACILLUS CEREUS FOOD POISONING

ID/CC	A **30-year-old female** presents to the surgical ER complaining of a stabbing **right upper quadrant abdominal pain.**
HPI	She is a prostitute who has been receiving treatment for **gonococcal pelvic inflammatory disease.**
PE	Right upper quadrant tenderness; mucopurulent cervicitis found on pelvic exam.
Labs	Cervical swab staining and culture identifies *Neisseria gonorrhoeae.*
Imaging	US: no evidence of cholecystitis. Peritoneoscopy: presence of "violin string" adhesions between liver capsule and peritoneum.
Gross Pathology	Adhesions noted between liver capsule and peritoneum.
Micro Pathology	N/A
Treatment	Antibiotic therapy (ceftriaxone and doxycycline).
Discussion	**Acute fibrinous perihepatitis** (= FITZ–HUGH–CURTIS SYNDROME) occurs as a complication of **gonococcal and chlamydial pelvic inflammatory disease** and clinically mimics cholecystitis.

FITZ–HUGH–CURTIS SYNDROME

ID/CC	A 25-year-old male complains of **midepigastric pain** that usually begins **1–2 hours after eating** and that occasionally awakens him at night.
HPI	The patient has been diagnosed with **duodenal ulcers** several times in the past, but his **symptoms have** consistently **recurred** even after therapy with H$_2$ blockers, antacids, and sucralfate.
PE	VS: stable. PE: pallor; epigastric tenderness on deep palpation.
Labs	CBC: normocytic, normochromic anemia. Stool positive for occult blood.
Imaging	Upper GI: ulcerations in antrum of stomach and duodenum; antral biopsy specimens yield **positive urease test.**
Gross Pathology	Grossly round ulcer (may also be oval) seen as sharply punched-out defect with relatively straight walls and slight overhanging of mucosal margin (heaped-up margin is characteristic of a malignant lesion); smooth and clean ulcer base.
Micro Pathology	No evidence of malignancy; **antral biopsies** reveal presence of **chronic mucosal inflammation.**
Treatment	Triple therapy with amoxicillin, metronidazole, and bismuth subsalicylate; triple therapy with clarithromycin, omeprazole, and tinidazole is now considered effective and relatively free of side effects.
Discussion	*H. pylori* grows overlying the antral gastric mucosal cells; 40% of healthy individuals and approximately 50% of patients with peptic disease harbor this organism. Although *H. pylori* **does not breach the epithelial barrier,** colonization of the antral mucosal layer by this organism is associated with structural alterations of the gastric mucosa and hence with a high prevalence of antral gastritis. Despite the fact that *H. pylori* does not grow on duodenal mucosa, it is strongly associated with duodenal ulcer, and eradication of the organism in patients with refractory peptic ulcer disease decreases the risk of recurrence. **FIRST AID** p.184

ID/CC	A 20-year-old male presents with an extensive **purpuric skin rash, oliguria,** and marked weakness; he also complains of **bloody diarrhea** of one week's duration.
HPI	The patient ate **a hamburger** at a fast-food restaurant 2–3 **days prior to the onset** of his diarrhea. He has no associated fever.
PE	VS: no fever. PE: dehydration; pallor; extensive purpuric skin rash.
Labs	Stool examination reveals presence of RBCs but **no inflammatory cells** or parasites; culture isolates sorbitol-negative *E. coli;* serotyping studies and effect on HeLa cell culture reveals presence of **enterohemorrhagic *E. coli* (EHEC) serotype O157:H7;** elevated BUN and creatinine. CBC/PBS: **microangiopathic anemia** and thrombocytopenia. PT, PTT normal.
Imaging	Sigmoidoscopy: moderately hyperemic mucosa with no evidence of any ulceration.
Gross Pathology	N/A
Micro Pathology	Pathology localized to kidney, where hyaline **thrombi** were seen **in afferent arterioles** and glomerular capillaries.
Treatment	Dialysis and blood transfusion for management of HUS; fluid and electrolyte maintenance; antimicrobial therapy. Most patients who develop HUS as a complication of *E. coli* hemorrhagic colitis die as a result of hemorrhagic complications.
Discussion	Hemorrhagic colitis associated with a Shiga-like toxin producing **EHEC O157:H7** is characterized by grossly bloody diarrhea with remarkably little fever or inflammatory exudate in stool; a significant number of patients develop potentially fatal HUS. EHEC infections can be largely **prevented through adequate cooking of beef,** especially hamburgers.

HEMORRHAGIC COLITIS WITH HEMOLYTIC–UREMIC SYNDROME (HUS)

ID/CC	A 28-year-old male from **India** complains of gradual-onset, intermittent, **crampy abdominal pain** with 1–4 **foul-smelling, frothy loose stools daily.**
HPI	His stools sometimes contain blood and mucus. He also complains of flatulence, tenesmus, and, at times, alternating diarrhea and constipation.
PE	Slight tenderness during palpation of cecum and ascending colon; no hepatomegaly.
Labs	CBC: mild leukocytosis; no eosinophilia. Fresh stool examination reveals presence of *Entamoeba histolytica* **cysts and motile hematophagous trophozoites;** serology for antiamebic antibodies is positive.
Imaging	Colonoscopy: **multiple colonic mucosal ulcers** that are slightly raised and covered with shaggy exudate; mucosa between ulcers normal.
Gross Pathology	N/A
Micro Pathology	Biopsy specimens reveal lesions extending under adjacent intact mucosa to produce classical **"flask-shaped" ulcers;** amebic trophozoites demonstrated at base of ulcer.
Treatment	**Metronidazole** (drug of choice) and diloxanide furoate or tetracycline.
Discussion	*Entamoeba histolytica* cysts are infective and are transmitted through contaminated water, raw vegetables, food handlers, and fecal–oral or oral–anal contact. The sites of involvement, in order of frequency, are the cecum and ascending colon, rectum, sigmoid colon, appendix, and terminal ileum. Complications include perforation of the bowel; liver abscess with pleural, pericardial, or peritoneal rupture; bowel obstruction by ameboma; and skin ulcers around the perineum and genitalia. **FIRST AID** p.193

INTESTINAL AMEBIASIS

ID/CC	A 14-year-old **malnourished child** died soon after hospitalization due to an **extensive small bowel rupture and shock.**
HPI	He had presented to the emergency room with **massive bloody diarrhea.** His history at admission revealed the presence of abdominal pain, fever, and diarrhea of a few days' duration; his symptoms had developed **after he ate leftover meat** at a fast-food restaurant.
PE	He was dehydrated, pale, and hypotensive at time of admission and developed signs of peritonitis and shock shortly before his death.
Labs	Culture and exam of necrotizing intestinal lesions isolated *Clostridium perfringens* **type C** producing beta toxin.
Imaging	N/A
Gross Pathology	Autopsy revealed ruptured small intestine, mucosal ulcerations, and **gas production** in the wall.
Micro Pathology	Microscopic exam revealed necrosis and acute inflammation in the ileum.
Treatment	Patient died despite aggressive fluid and electrolyte replacement, bowel decompression, and antibiotic therapy (penicillin, chloramphenicol); surgery had been planned in view of rupture of the small bowel
Discussion	Necrotizing enterocolitis is a condition affecting poorly nourished persons who suddenly feast on meat (pigbel). It is associated with *Clostridium perfringens* **type C** and **beta enterotoxin;** beta toxin paralyzes the villi and causes friability and necrosis of the bowel wall. Immunization of children in New Guinea with beta-toxoid vaccine has dramatically decreased the incidence of the disease.

· ·

NECROTIZING ENTEROCOLITIS

ID/CC	A 7-year-old male who has been hospitalized for treatment of **acute lymphocytic leukemia** complains of **copious watery diarrhea**, right lower quadrant **abdominal pain**, and **fever**.
HPI	He was diagnosed as **neutropenic** (due to aggressive cytotoxic chemotherapy) a few days ago.
PE	VS: fever; tachycardia; tachypnea. PE: pallor; sternal tenderness; axillary lymphadenopathy; hepatosplenomegaly; abdominal distention; moderate dehydration.
Labs	CBC: severe **neutropenia**; anemia; thrombocytopenia. PBS and bone marrow studies suggest he is in remission; blood culture grows microaerophilic *Clostridium septicum.*
Imaging	CT-Abdomen: **thickening of cecal wall.**
Gross Pathology	Mucosal ulcers and inflammation in **ileocecal region** of small intestine.
Micro Pathology	N/A
Treatment	Aggressive **supportive measures**; surgical intervention; appropriate **antibiotics**.
Discussion	Neutropenic enterocolitis is a fulminant form of necrotizing enteritis that occurs in neutropenic patients; neutropenia is often related to cyclic neutropenia, leukemia, aplastic anemia, or chemotherapy. In postmortem exams of patients who have died of leukemia, infections of the cecal area (= TYPHLITIS) are frequently found; *C. septicum* is the most common organism isolated from the blood of such patients.

· ·

NEUTROPENIC ENTEROCOLITIS

ID/CC	A **4-year-old** male is brought to the physician by his parents, who complain that the child has had **intense perianal itching**, especially **during the night**.
HPI	The child is otherwise healthy, and his developmental progress is normal.
PE	Perianal excoriation noted.
Labs	Cellulose adhesive tape secured to perianal area during the night reveals presence of *Enterobius vermicularis* eggs that were **flattened on one side, were embryonated, and had a thick shell**; no parasites found on stool exam.
Imaging	N/A
Gross Pathology	N/A
Micro Pathology	N/A
Treatment	Strict **personal hygiene**; drugs used include **mebendazole, piperazine,** and **pyrantel pamoate**.
Discussion	Infection is caused by *Enterobius vermicularis*. Adult worms are located primarily in the cecal region; **female adult worms migrate to the perianal area during the night and deposit their eggs**. Direct person-to-person **infection occurs by** ingestion and **swallowing of eggs; autoinoculation** occurs by contamination of fingers. The life cycle is completed in about six weeks.

· ·

PINWORM INFECTION

ID/CC	A 30-year-old **hospitalized** male presents with **profuse watery diarrhea with mucus,** crampy periumbilical **abdominal pain,** nausea, and vomiting.
HPI	He has been receiving **oral ampicillin** for five days for a lower respiratory tract infection.
PE	VS: fever; tachycardia. PE: dehydration; abdominal distention; diffuse rebound tenderness; reduced bowel sounds.
Labs	CBC: leukocytosis (15,000/uL) with predominantly polymorphonuclear leukocytosis. Fecal staining reveals few RBCs and leukocytes (< 10 cells/HPF); *Clostridium difficile* toxin A in stool demonstrated by ELISA.
Imaging	Sigmoidoscopy: erythematous colonic mucosa with edema; yellowish plaques with erythematous border.
Gross Pathology	Patchy areas of black material containing mucus, fibrin, inflammatory cells, and necrotic debris attached to a diffusely hyperemic border.
Micro Pathology	Exudative punctate, raised plaques (= PSEUDOMEMBRANES) with edematous, hyperemic mucosa on biopsy; crypt abscesses; thrombosis of submucosal venules.
Treatment	**Discontinue antibiotics** (ampicillin); fluid and electrolyte replacement; **metronidazole, vancomycin** (less preferable because vancomycin can select for vancomycin-resistant enterococci).
Discussion	Pseudomembranous colitis (PMC) is a **toxin-mediated inflammatory process** that is characterized by exudative plaques or pseudomembranes attached to the surface of inflamed mucosa. The most frequently implicated antimicrobials in PMC are **ampicillin, clindamycin, and cephalosporins.**

· ·

PSEUDOMEMBRANOUS COLITIS

ID/CC	A **10-month-old** male presents with fever and severe **vomiting** followed by **watery diarrhea.**
HPI	His stools are loose and watery without blood or mucus.
PE	VS: fever; tachycardia. PE: child is irritable; moderate dehydration.
Labs	Absence of leukocytes on fecal stain; rotavirus detected with **ELISA; electron microscopy** with negative staining identifies **rotavirus** on stool ultrafiltrates.
Imaging	N/A
Gross Pathology	N/A
Micro Pathology	Major histopathologic lesions are characterized by reversible involvement of the proximal small intestine; mucosa remains intact with shortening of villi, a mixed inflammatory infiltration of lamina propria, and hyperplasia of the mucosal crypt cells; electron microscopy reveals distended cisterns of endoplasmic reticulum, mitochondrial swelling, and sparse, irregular microvilli.
Treatment	**Fluid replacement therapy.**
Discussion	Rotavirus group A is the single **most important cause** of endemic, **severe diarrheal illness in infants and young children worldwide;** it occurs with greater frequency during winter months in temperate climates and during the dry season in tropical climates. In the United States, rotavirus accounts for 50% of all childhood diarrheas, has an incubation period of 48 hours, is transmitted by the fecal–oral route, and lasts only a few days. Some children subsequently develop lactose intolerance, which lasts for a few weeks.

ID/CC	A 30-year-old male presents with sudden-onset, crampy **abdominal pain and diarrhea.**
HPI	The diarrhea is watery and contains mucus. The patient also complains of low-grade fever with chills, malaise, nausea, and vomiting. Careful history reveals that he had ingested **partially cooked eggs** at a poultry farm 24 hours before his symptoms began.
PE	VS: fever; tachycardia. PE: mild diffuse abdominal tenderness; mild dehydration.
Labs	Stool culture yields *Salmonella typhimurium;* stained stool demonstrates PMNs.
Imaging	N/A
Gross Pathology	Intestinal mucosal erythema (limited to the colon) and some superficial ulcers.
Micro Pathology	Mixed inflammatory infiltrate in mucosa; superficial epithelial erosions.
Treatment	Fluid and electrolyte replacement therapy; **antibiotics** withheld, as they **prolong carrier state.** Antibiotic therapy only for malnourished, severely ill, suspected bacteremia, and sickle cell disease.
Discussion	Infection is acquired through the ingestion of food (**eggs, meat, poultry**) or water contaminated with animal or human feces; individuals with **low gastric acidity** are also susceptible. **FIRST AID** p.184

SALMONELLA FOOD POISONING

ID/CC	A 25-year-old male presents with sudden-onset, severe **vomiting**, nausea, **abdominal cramps, and diarrhea.**
HPI	He had returned home about two hours after attending a birthday party at which **meat and milk** were served in various forms. The **friend** who was celebrating his birthday **reported similar symptoms.**
PE	VS: no fever. PE: mild dehydration; diffuse abdominal tenderness; increased bowel sounds.
Labs	**Toxigenic staphylococcus** recovered from culturing food. Coagulase-positive staphylococcus cultured from **nose of one of the cooks** at party.
Imaging	N/A
Gross Pathology	N/A
Micro Pathology	No mucosal lesions.
Treatment	Fluid and electrolyte balance; antibiotics not indicated.
Discussion	*Staphylococcus aureus* food poisoning results from the ingestion of food containing **preformed heat-stable enterotoxin B.** Outbreaks of staphylococcal food poisoning occur when food handlers who have contaminated superficial wounds or who are shedding infected nasal droplets inoculate foods such as meat, dairy products, salad dressings, cream sauces, and custard-filled pastries. The **incubation period** ranges from **two to eight hours;** the disease is self-limited.

· ·

STAPHYLOCOCCUS AUREUS GASTROENTERITIS

ID/CC	A 25-year-old male U.S. citizen on **vacation in Mexico** presents with abrupt-onset **watery diarrhea, abdominal cramps,** and a **low-grade fever** and chills.
HPI	The patient does not complain of tenesmus or passage of blood or mucus in his stools, but he does complain of a feeling of urgency to defecate.
PE	VS: low-grade fever. PE: unremarkable.
Labs	No erythrocytes, WBCs, or parasites seen in stained stool; bioassays for enterotoxigenic *E. coli* (ETEC) reveal presence of the labile **enterotoxin (LT)** (tests available only for research purposes).
Imaging	N/A
Gross Pathology	N/A
Micro Pathology	N/A
Treatment	Fluid replacement; antibiotics (cotrimoxazole, quinolones); prevention with careful hygienic practices and prophylactic daily doxycycline.
Discussion	Traveler's diarrhea is a self-limited condition that is most often due to ingestion of contaminated food or drinks. Over three-fourths of cases of traveler's diarrhea are caused by bacteria, with enterotoxigenic *E. coli* the most frequent cause (may also be caused by enteropathogenic *E. coli* and, in Mexico, by an enteroadherent *E. coli*). Other common pathogens include *Shigella* species, *Campylobacter jejuni,* *Aeromonas* species, *Plesiomonas shigelloides,* *Salmonella* species, and noncholera vibrios. Rotavirus and Norwalk agent are the most common viral causes; *Giardia,* *Cryptosporidium,* and, rarely, *Entamoeba histolytica* are parasitic pathogens. Enterotoxigenic *E. coli* produce enterotoxins that bind to intestinal receptors and **activate adenyl cyclase** in the intestinal cell to produce an increase in the level of the cyclic nucleotides cAMP (LT, labile toxin) and cGMP (ST, stable toxin), which markedly augments sodium, chloride, and water loss, thereby producing a **secretory diarrhea.**

· ·

TRAVELER'S DIARRHEA

ID/CC	A 30-year-old male presents with sudden-onset fever, colicky **abdominal pain**, and **watery diarrhea.**
HPI	He had eaten **crabs** at a friend's party the day before (incubation period 16–48 hours).
PE	VS: fever; tachycardia. PE: no dehydration; diffuse abdominal tenderness; increased bowel sounds.
Labs	*Vibrio parahaemolyticus* isolated from stool in a high-salt-content (halophilic vibrio) culture medium; PMNs in stool; **Kanagawa phenomenon** (beta-hemolysis on medium containing human blood; done as an indicator for pathogenicity) **positive.**
Imaging	N/A
Gross Pathology	N/A
Micro Pathology	N/A
Treatment	Fluid and electrolyte balance; antibiotics not required.
Discussion	**Seafood** is the main source of the organism. After ingestion, *Vibrio parahaemolyticus* multiplies in the gut and produces a **diarrheal enterotoxin.**

ID/CC	A 35-year-old male presents to the emergency room with high-grade fever, marked weakness, and a **vesiculobullous skin eruption.**
HPI	He had just returned from the Gulf of Mexico, where he had consumed large quantities of **seafood.** He has been diagnosed with **chronic liver disease** (due to hemochromatosis).
PE	VS: fever; hypotension; tachycardia. PE: icterus; vesiculobullous skin lesions seen on an otherwise-bronzed complexion.
Labs	Hyperglycemia; blood culture on **high-salt medium** (halophilic bacteria) reveals growth of *Vibrio vulnificus;* evidence of hemochromatosis (hyperglycemia, hyperbilirubinemia, increased serum iron).
Imaging	N/A
Gross Pathology	N/A
Micro Pathology	N/A
Treatment	Tetracycline, ciprofloxacin; supportive.
Discussion	Halophilic *Vibrio vulnificus* should be suspected and treated in any individual with chronic liver disease who presents with septicemia and skin lesions 1–3 days following seafood ingestion.

· ·

VIBRIO VULNIFICUS FOOD POISONING

ID/CC An 8-year-old male is brought to a physician with complaints of **impairment of vision** in the left eye, **urticarial skin rashes**, and ill-defined muscle aches.

HPI The child's mother has caught the child eating dirt or soil on many occasions (= PICA). The family also has a **pet dog** at home.

PE **Rounded swelling near the optic disc** seen on fundus exam of left eye; **urticarial wheals** observed on extremities and trunk; mild **hepatosplenomegaly** noted.

Labs Leukocytosis with marked **eosinophilia**; enzyme immunoassay using extracts of excretory-secretory products of *Toxocara canis* larvae positive.

Imaging N/A

Gross Pathology N/A

Micro Pathology Biopsy of liver reveals larvae with granuloma and eosinophilic infiltration.

Treatment **Thiabendazole**; steroids to control inflammatory response; laser photocoagulation of visible ocular larvae.

Discussion When the nondefinitive human host is infected with parasites that normally infect animals, the parasites do not mature completely, but the larvae introduced persist and induce an inflammatory reaction. The syndrome of **visceral larva migrans** develops when nematode larvae of animal parasites (**mostly cat or dog ascarids** such as *T. canis*) migrate in human tissues; the syndrome of **cutaneous larva migrans** (creeping eruption) develops when the larvae of various parasites (including the **dog or cat hookworm** *Ancylostoma braziliense*) penetrate human skin and form pruritic, serpiginous cutaneous lesions along the migratory tracts of the larvae.

. . . .

VISCERAL LARVA MIGRANS

ID/CC	A 28-year-old female complains of **painful swelling of both knees** and **tender skin eruptions** on both shins.
HPI	For the past two weeks she has also had **watery diarrhea** that developed after she consumed some **raw pork.** She also complains of low-grade fever and mild abdominal pain.
PE	VS: low-grade fever; tachycardia. PE: mild dehydration; swollen and warm knee joints with painful restriction of all movements (= ARTHRITIS); multiple, **tender, erythematous plaques and nodules** (= ERYTHEMA NODOSUM) seen over both shins.
Labs	CBC: leukocytosis. *Yersinia enterocolitica* isolated from stool; patient is **HLA-B27 positive.**
Imaging	N/A
Gross Pathology	N/A
Micro Pathology	Oval ulcers with long axis in the direction of bowel flow, similar to ulcers caused by typhoid fever(intestinal tubercular ulcers are transverse).
Treatment	Supportive; antibiotics (aminoglycosides, fluoroquinolones) indicated in severe infections.
Discussion	*Yersinia enterocolitica* is an **intracellular pathogen** that causes **gastroenteritis,** most frequently involving the distal ileum and colon (enterotoxin mediated), **mesenteric adenitis** (due to necrotizing and suppurative gut lesions) and ileitis (pseudoappendicitis), and sepsis; infection may trigger a variety of **autoimmune phenomena,** including erythema nodosum, reactive arthritis, and possibly thyroiditis, especially in HLA-B27-positive individuals.

YERSINIA ENTEROCOLITIS

ID/CC	A **4-month-old male** presents with **chronic diarrhea** and **failure to thrive**.
HPI	The infant was diagnosed with extensive **mucocutaneous candidiasis** in the early neonatal period and shortly thereafter developed a fulminant *Pseudomonas* **septicemia** that required intravenous antibiotic therapy for an extended period of time. A paternal cousin had developed similar and equally devastating bacterial and fungal infections in the neonatal period and subsequently died.
PE	Emaciated; mucocutaneous **candidiasis** noted; **tonsils not seen; lymph nodes not palpable** despite recurrent infections.
Labs	CBC: severe lymphopenia. PBS: **lack of mature lymphocytes.** Tests for cutaneous **delayed hypersensitivity** and contact sensitization negative; **serum immunoglobulin levels (IgG, IgA, and IgM) low; adenosine deaminase (ADA) deficiency** demonstrated in red cells.
Imaging	CXR: **absent thymic shadow.**
Gross Pathology	Thymus fails to descend into the anterior mediastinum from the neck and resembles fetal thymus of 6–8 weeks.
Micro Pathology	No lymphoid tissue in the lymph nodes, spleen, tonsils, and appendix.
Treatment	**Bone marrow transplant** from an HLA-identical sibling; IV immunoglobulin; infusion of normal ADA-containing erythrocytes (ADA-PEG is also very successful); antibiotics; gene therapy for ADA; genetic counseling (SCID caused by ADA deficiency can be diagnosed prenatally by amniocentesis).
Discussion	Severe combined immunodeficiency syndrome is characterized by marked depletion of the cells that mediate both humoral (B-cell) and cellular (T-cell) immunity. SCID may be transmitted as either an autosomal-recessive trait or an X-linked recessive trait, or it may be sporadic; half of the cases inherited in an **autosomal-recessive** manner are caused by a **deficiency in ADA.** **FIRST AID** p.209

. . . .

SEVERE COMBINED IMMUNODEFICIENCY SYNDROME (SCID)

ID/CC	A 10-year-old male complains of generalized weakness, faintness on exertion, and occasional epigastric pain
HPI	His mother has noticed that he often **eats soil and other inedible things** (= PICA).
PE	Pallor; puffy face and dependent edema.
Labs	CBC: **microcytic, hypochromic anemia; eosinophilia. Low serum iron and ferritin;** elevated serum transferrin; reduced bone marrow hemosiderin; **hypoproteinemia;** stool exam revealed **eggs of *Ancylostoma duodenale*** (ovoid eggs with thin transparent shell that reveal the segmented embryo within).
Imaging	N/A
Gross Pathology	N/A
Micro Pathology	N/A
Treatment	**Albendazole** or mebendazole; **iron supplementation** to treat iron deficiency anemia.
Discussion	Infection with hookworms, either *Ancylostoma duodenale* or *Necator americanus,* is more likely where insanitary conditions exist; individuals at risk include children, gardeners, plumbers or electricians who are in contact with soil, and armed-forces personnel. Hookworm eggs excreted in the feces hatch in the soil, releasing larvae that develop into infective larvae. Percutaneous larval penetration is the principal mode of human infection. From the skin, hookworm larvae travel via the bloodstream to the lungs, enter the alveoli, ascend the bronchotracheal tree to the pharynx, and are swallowed. Although transpulmonary larval passage may elicit a transient **eosinophilic pneumonitis** (= LÖFFLER'S PNEUMONITIS), this phenomenon is much less common with hookworm infections than with roundworm infections. The major health impact of hookworm infection, however, is iron loss resulting from the 0.1–0.4 ml of blood ingested daily by each adult worm. In malnourished hosts, such blood loss can lead to **severe iron deficiency anemia.**

· ·

HOOKWORM

ID/CC A 30-year-old female presents to the ER with **severe, sudden-onset shortness of breath** and an **extensive** pruritic **skin rash.**

HPI She was **prescribed cotrimoxazole** by her general physician for a UTI; she took the **first dose only a few minutes before** developing symptoms.

PE VS: **hypotension.** PE: severe **respiratory distress;** central cyanosis; extensive **urticarial wheals** noted all over body.

Labs **IgE antibody** demonstrated to sulfonamides by **RAST.**

Imaging N/A

Gross Pathology N/A

Micro Pathology N/A

Treatment **Epinephrine** (1:1000); antihistaminics; steroids; ventilatory support; adequate intravenous fluid administration or vasopressor agents to treat hypotension.

Discussion Systemic anaphylaxis is the most serious and life-threatening **IgE-mediated type 1 hypersensitivity reaction;** its recognition and prompt treatment are critical to survival.

ANAPHYLACTIC REACTION

ID/CC	A 35-year-old **Finnish** man complains of **easy fatigability and shortness of breath.**
HPI	He often eats **undercooked or raw freshwater fish.** He also reports vague digestive disturbances such as anorexia, heartburn, and nausea.
PE	PE: pallor.
Labs	CBC/PBS: **megaloblastic anemia.** Blood **vitamin B$_{12}$ levels low;** stool exam reveals presence of **operculated eggs and proglottids of** *D. latum.*
Imaging	N/A
Gross Pathology	N/A
Micro Pathology	N/A
Treatment	Niclosamide or praziquantel.
Discussion	*Diphyllobothrium latum* infection is found in cold climates where **raw or undercooked fish** are eaten. The adult worm attaches to the human jejunum and **competes for absorption of vitamin B$_{12}$,** producing a deficiency that resembles pernicious anemia.

· ·

ANEMIA WITH DIPHYLLOBOTHRIUM LATUM INFECTION

ID/CC	A 45-year-old male with refractory **acute myeloid leukemia** who underwent a **bone marrow transplant** from a nonidentical donor presents with an **extensive skin rash**, severe **diarrhea**, and **jaundice**.
HPI	Prior to the transplant, which occurred two months ago, he **received preparative chemotherapy and radiotherapy** along with broad-spectrum antibiotics. Engraftment was confirmed within four weeks by rising leukocyte counts.
PE	VS: normotension. PE: patient is cachectic and moderately dehydrated; icterus noted; violaceous, scaly macules and erythematous papules **resembling lichen planus** seen over extremities.
Labs	CBC: falling blood counts; relative eosinophilia. Elevated direct serum bilirubin and transaminases; stool exam reveals no infectious etiology; skin biopsy taken.
Imaging	N/A
Gross Pathology	Skin biopsy specimens reveal vacuolar changes of basal cell layer with perivenular lymphocytic infiltrates (CD8+ T cells).
Micro Pathology	N/A
Treatment	**High-dose cyclosporine therapy**, rabbit anti-thymocyte globulin, methylprednisolone or anti-T-cell monoclonal antibodies.
Discussion	Approximately 30% of bone marrow transplant recipients develop graft-versus-host disease (GVHD). This attack is primarily launched by immunocompetent T lymphocytes derived from the donor's marrow against the cells and tissues of the recipient, which it recognizes as foreign. Cyclosporin A is effective for prevention of GVHD.

GRAFT-VERSUS-HOST DISEASE

ID/CC	An **8-year-old child** with **sickle cell anemia** is seen with complaints of sudden-onset **pallor of the skin** and mucous membranes, fatigue, and malaise.
HPI	The child suffered a **mild prodromal illness** before developing severe pallor.
PE	VS: no fever; tachycardia; tachypnea; normotension. PE: severe pallor; mild icterus; no lymphadenopathy, splenomegaly, or hepatomegaly noted.
Labs	CBC: **severe anemia** (Hb 2 gm/dL); **reduced leukocyte** and platelet counts; mild hyperbilirubinemia; **absent reticulocytes** and sickled RBCs on peripheral blood smear.
Imaging	N/A
Gross Pathology	N/A
Micro Pathology	Bone marrow biopsy reveals increased numbers of **giant pronormoblasts** (diagnostic of parvovirus infection).
Treatment	Blood transfusions to tide over the crises. Spontaneous recovery in 1–2 weeks.
Discussion	Parvovirus infection is the cause of **transient aplastic crises** (may also be due to folic acid deficiency) that occur in patients who have severe **hemolytic disorders;** cessation of erythropoiesis for about 10 days in a normal adult as a result of parvovirus infection would produce a 10% drop in hemoglobin concentration (i.e., a fall of 1% daily would lead to a decline in hemoglobin concentration of 1–2 g/dL after 10 days). A patient with severe hemolysis in whom the bone marrow is turning over at a rate seven times normal would experience a 70% decrease in hemoglobin concentration (i.e., a drop from 10 g/dL to 3 g/dL) as a result of a 10-day cessation of erythropoiesis. Although parvovirus can affect all precursor cells, the red cell precursors are most profoundly affected.

. . . .

PARVOVIRUS B19 (APLASTIC CRISIS)

ID/CC	A 34-year-old male presents to his primary care physician with a hard, red, painless **swelling** on his left **mandible** that has slowly been growing over the past few weeks and has now begun to **drain pus.**
HPI	The patient **recently had a tooth extraction.**
PE	No acute distress; no other significant findings.
Labs	Gram stain of exudate reveals **branching gram-positive filaments** and characteristic **"sulfur granules"**; non-acid-fast and anaerobic (distinguishes actinomyces from *Nocardia*).
Imaging	XR: no bony destruction.
Gross Pathology	**Sinus tracts** from region of infection to surface with granular exudate.
Micro Pathology	Granulation tissue and fibrosis surrounding a central suppurative necrosis; granulation tissue may also enclose foamy histiocytes and plasma cells.
Treatment	Penicillin G followed by oral penicillin V and, if necessary, surgical drainage and removal of necrotic tissue.
Discussion	*Actinomyces israelii* is a part of the normal flora of the mouth (crypts of tonsils and tartar of teeth), so most patients have a history of surgery or trauma. There is **no person-to-person spread.** Actinomycosis is a chronic suppurative infection and can also involve the abdomen or lungs, especially following a penetrating trauma such as a bullet wound or an intestinal perforation. Pelvic disease is associated with IUD use. Spread occurs contiguously, not hematogenously. **FIRST AID** p.174

ACTINOMYCOSIS

ID/CC	A 6-year-old male presents with complaints of a **mild sore throat and eye irritation.**
HPI	His mother says that he has spent hours at the **community swimming pool** this summer.
PE	Mild **rhinopharyngitis;** bilateral **conjunctival congestion** with scanty mucoid discharge.
Labs	Viral culture of conjunctival and nasopharyngeal swab yields **adenovirus.**
Imaging	N/A
Gross Pathology	N/A
Micro Pathology	N/A
Treatment	No specific treatment; self-limiting illness.
Discussion	Adenovirus infections occur most often in **infants and young children,** who acquire the virus by the **respiratory or fecal–oral** route. The most common respiratory tract syndrome in this age group is mild coryza with pharyngitis; in older children, these symptoms may be accompanied by conjunctivitis. On electron microscopy it is seen as a **double-stranded nonenveloped DNA virus** surrounded by a 20-faced icosahedral protein capsid from which 12 antenna-like fibers or pentons extend radially. **FIRST AID** p.197

ADENOVIRUS PHARYNGITIS

ID/CC	A 28-year-old **male homosexual** complains of continuous low-grade **fever, weight loss,** and **diarrhea** of one month's duration.
HPI	He also complains of an **extensive skin rash, mucous membrane eruptions, recurrent herpes zoster infection,** and **oral ulcerations.** He reports practicing receptive anal intercourse.
PE	VS: low-grade fever. PS: cachectic; **generalized lymphadenopathy;** maculopapular rash; severe **seborrheic dermatitis; oral thrush;** white confluent patch with corrugated surface (= ORAL HAIRY LEUKOPLAKIA) along lateral borders of tongue; **penile warts** (= CONDYLOMATA ACUMINATA); extensive multiple pruritic, pink, umbilicated papules 2–5 mm in diameter (= MOLLUSCUM CONTAGIOSUM).
Labs	CBC: anemia; leukopenia with lymphopenia; thrombocytopenia. **Low CD4+ count;** elevated CD8+ T-cell count; ELISA for HIV-1 positive; **Western blot confirmatory; PCR for viral RNA** (investigation of choice in window period) **positive.**
Imaging	N/A
Gross Pathology	N/A
Micro Pathology	**Oral hairy leukoplakia;** lesions show keratin projections resembling hairs, koilocytosis, and little atypia; hybridization techniques reveal **Epstein–Barr virus** in lesions.
Treatment	Prophylactic antibiotics for prevention of opportunistic infections while monitoring CD4+ T-cell counts; antiretroviral drugs (zidovudine, didanosine, zalcitabine, and protease inhibitors); counseling and rehabilitative measures.
Discussion	AIDS-related complex (ARC) consists of symptomatic conditions in an HIV-infected patient that are not included in the AIDS surveillance case definition and that meet at least one of the following criteria: (1) the conditions are indicative of a defect in cell-mediated immunity; or (2) the conditions have a clinical course or management that is complicated by HIV infection.

. . . .

AIDS-RELATED COMPLEX (ARC)

ID/CC	A 50-year-old male presents to the ER with complaints of **recurrent,** sudden-onset, **severe breathlessness,** wheezing, fever, chills, and a **productive cough** (sometimes producing **brown bronchial casts**).
HPI	The patient has had steroid-dependent **chronic bronchial asthma** for many years and has no history of foreign travel or contact with a TB patient. He has a history of **occasional hemoptysis.**
PE	VS: fever; marked tachycardia; severe tachypnea. PE: respiratory distress; central cyanosis; wheezing; rhonchi and coarse rales over both lung fields.
Labs	CBC: **eosinophilia.** Oxygen saturation low. Very high titers of specific **IgE antibodies against** *Aspergillus* present (specific marker for the disease); sputum cultures positive for *Aspergillus;* **skin tests** to *Aspergillus* antigens **positive.** PFTs: obstructive picture (due to underlying asthma).
Imaging	CXR: **segmental infiltrate** in upper lobes (these infiltrates are segmental because they correspond directly to the affected bronchi); **branching, fingerlike shadows** from mucoid impaction of dilated central bronchi (virtually **pathognomonic** of allergic bronchopulmonary aspergillosis). CT-Chest: evidence of **proximal bronchiectasis.**
Gross Pathology	N/A
Micro Pathology	N/A
Treatment	Oral corticosteroids or beclomethasone.
Discussion	Allergic bronchopulmonary aspergillosis (ABPA) is a hypersensitivity disorder that primarily affects the central bronchi; immediate and Arthus-type hypersensitivity reactions are involved in its pathogenesis. The onset of the disease occurs most often in the fourth and fifth decades, and virtually all patients have long-standing atopic asthma. Untreated ABPA leads to proximal bronchiectasis. FIRST AID p.189

. . . .

ALLERGIC BRONCHOPULMONARY ASPERGILLOSIS

ID/CC	A 50-year-old **alcoholic male** presents with a high-grade **fever, cough, copious, foul-smelling sputum,** and pleuritic right-sided chest pain.
HPI	His wife reports that he was brought home in a **semiconscious state a few days ago,** when he was found lying on the roadside heavily under the influence of alcohol.
PE	VS: fever. PE: signs of consolidation elicited over **right middle and lower pulmonary lobes.**
Labs	Sputum reveals abundant PMN leukocytes and mixed oral flora; **culture yields *B. melaninogenicus (Prevotella melaninogenica)* and other *Bacteroides* species,** *Fusobacterium,* **microaerophilic streptococci,** and *Peptostreptococcus.*
Imaging	CXR: **consolidation involving apical segment of right lower lobe and posterior segments of middle lobe;** large cavity with air–fluid level (= ABSCESS) also seen.
Gross Pathology	N/A
Micro Pathology	N/A
Treatment	**Clindamycin.**
Discussion	Alcoholism, drug abuse, administration of sedatives or anesthesia, head trauma, and seizures or other neurologic disorders are most often responsible for the development of aspiration pneumonia. Because anaerobes are the dominant flora of the upper respiratory tract (outnumbering aerobic or facultative bacteria by 10 to 1), they are the dominant organisms in aspiration pneumonia; of particular importance are *Bacteroides melaninogenicus (Prevotella melaninogenica)* and other *Bacteroides* species (slender, pleomorphic, pale gram-negative rods), *Fusobacterium nucleatum* (slender gram-negative rods with pointed ends), and anaerobic or microaerophilic streptococci and *Peptostreptococcus* (small gram-positive cocci in chains or clumps).

. . . .

ASPIRATION PNEUMONIA WITH LUNG ABSCESS

ID/CC	A 38-year-old **HIV-positive** male is admitted to the hospital with **fever, rigors, night sweats, and diarrhea.**
HPI	He reports excessive weight loss over the past few weeks. He was treated for *Pneumocystis* pneumonia a few weeks ago and still reports a persistent productive cough.
PE	VS: fever. PE: patient is extremely emaciated; hepatosplenomegaly and lymphadenopathy noted.
Labs	CD4+ count < 50/cc; *Mycobacterium avium-intracellulare* isolated on blood culture; smears of tissues obtained from lymph nodes, bone marrow, spleen, liver, and lungs reveal evidence of acid-fast bacilli and cultures yield *M. avium;* intestinal infection with *M. avium* proven by culture of stools and colonic biopsy specimens.
Imaging	CT-Abd: hepatosplenomegaly, retroperitoneal lymphadenopathy, bowel mucosal fold thickening.
Gross Pathology	N/A
Micro Pathology	Despite the presence of many mycobacteria and macrophages, well-formed granulomas were typically absent due to **profound impairment of cell-mediated immunity.**
Treatment	Multidrug regimens comprising newer **macrolides, amikacin, ethambutol, clofazimine, rifampicin** (used for prophylaxis), and **quinolones.**
Discussion	*Mycobacterium avium* complex is now the **most frequent opportunistic bacterial infection in patients with AIDS**; it typically occurs late in the course of the syndrome, when other opportunistic infections and neoplasia have already occurred. Lifetime **prophylaxis with rifabutin** is recommended for AIDS patients whose CD4+ cell counts have fallen below 100/mm^3.

. . . .

ATYPICAL MYCOBACTERIAL INFECTION IN AIDS

ID/CC   A 30-year-old male who recently emigrated from **Peru** presents with an extensive **nodular skin eruption**, mild arthralgias, and occasional fever.

HPI   One month ago, the patient had a high-grade **fever** that was accompanied by excessive weakness, dyspnea, and passage of **cola-colored urine**; the fever subsided after two weeks, but his weakness has progressed since that time.

PE   Pallor; mild icterus; extensive skin rash comprising **purplish nodular lesions** of varying sizes seen on face, trunk, and limbs; mild hepatosplenomegaly; funduscopy reveals **retinal hemorrhages**.

Labs   **Intraerythrocytic coccobacillary**-form bacteria visible in thick and thin films stained with Giemsa; **bacteria** seen and **isolated from skin lesions**; indirect serum bilirubin elevated. PBS: macrocytic, hypochromic anemia with polychromasia; marked reticulocytosis (due to hemolytic anemia); Coombs' test negative.

Imaging   N/A

Gross Pathology   N/A

Micro Pathology   Skin biopsy of vascular skin lesions reveals endothelial proliferation and histiocytic hyperplasia; electron microscopy of verrucous tissue shows *Bartonella bacilliformis* in interstitial tissue.

Treatment   **Chloramphenicol, penicillin, erythromycin, norfloxacin,** and **tetracycline** are effective; rifampicin is indicated for treatment of verrucous forms

Discussion   Bartonellosis is a sandfly-borne bacterial disease occurring only on the **western coast of South America** at high altitudes; the causative agent is a motile, pleomorphic bacillus, *B. bacilliformis*. Two stages of the disease are recognized: an **initial febrile stage** associated with a **hemolytic anemia** (= OROYA FEVER) and a later cutaneous stage characterized by **hemangiomatous nodules** (= VERRUGA PERUANA).

· ·

BARTONELLOSIS

ID/CC	A 32-year-old male is referred to a tertiary care center with **chronic pneumonia** and **warty lesions** on his left upper limb.
HPI	The patient is from the **southeastern United States.** His skin lesions are nonpruritic and painless. He also complains of malaise, weight loss, night sweats, chest pain, breathlessness, and hoarseness.
PE	VS: fever; tachycardia; mild tachypnea. PE: **bilateral rales and rhonchi;** raised, **verrucous, and crusted lesions** with serpiginous border located on left upper extremity; small abscesses demonstrable when superficial crust was removed.
Labs	Sputum and pus from cutaneous lesions demonstrate **spherical cells** (8–15 mm in diameter) that have a **thick-walled, refractile double contour** and show unipolar (broad based) budding; culture of pus and sputum on Sabouraud's agar yields **growth of *Blastomyces;*** no evidence of acid-fast bacilli found either on staining or on culture; Gomori's methenamine silver staining of lung tissue does not reveal *Pneumocystis.*
Imaging	CXR: bilateral alveolar consolidations with air-bronchograms.
Gross Pathology	N/A
Micro Pathology	Epithelioid macrophages and giant cells surrounding a suppurative center; skin lesions show pseudoepitheliomatous hyperplasia very similar to squamous cell carcinoma.
Treatment	Itraconazole is treatment of choice in most patients; amphotericin B, fluconazole, and ketoconazole are alternative drugs.
Discussion	Blastomycosis is a systemic mycotic infection of humans and dogs that is characterized by suppuration and granulomatous lesions and is caused by the **dimorphic fungus *Blastomyces dermatitidis;*** the disease is **endemic in the southeastern and south-central portions of the United States,** and several pockets of infection extend north along the Mississippi and Ohio rivers into central Canada. Clinical disease most commonly involves the lungs (acquired by spore inhalation) and then, by hematogenous dissemination, the skin, the skeletal system, and the male genitourinary tract. **FIRST AID** p.188

. . . .

BLASTOMYCOSIS

ID/CC   A 26-year-old female presents to the ER with intense, acute-onset left **lower quadrant crampy abdominal pain,** foul-smelling stools with streaks of blood, urgency, **tenesmus,** and fever.

HPI   For the past two days, the patient has also had headaches and myalgias. She frequently **drinks unpasteurized** ("raw") **milk** that she buys at a health-food store.

PE   VS: fever (39 C); tachycardia; normal RR and BP. PE: no dehydration; diffuse abdominal tenderness more marked in left lower quadrant.

Labs   Stool smear shows leukocytes (due to invasive tissue damage in the colon) and **gram-negative, curved, bacilli,** often in pairs, in "gull-wing"-shaped pattern; dark-field exam shows motility; culture in microaerophilic, 42 C conditions on special agar yields *Campylobacter jejuni,* indicated by oxidase and catalase positivity.

Imaging   N/A.

Gross Pathology   Friable colonic mucosa.

Micro Pathology   Nonspecific inflammatory reaction consisting of neutrophils, lymphocytes and plasma cells with hyperemia, edema and damage to epithelium, glandular degeneration, ulcerations, and crypt abscesses caused by colonic tissue invasion of the organism.

Treatment   Self-limiting disease. Severe cases can be treated with aminoglycosides and erythromycin.

Discussion   One of the primary causes of "traveler's diarrhea." Sources of infection include **undercooked food** and contact with **infected animals** and their excreta. Prevent by improving public sanitation, pasteurizing milk, and proper cooking.

ID/CC	A 25-year-old female presents with **painful lumps in her right axilla** and neck together with **low-grade fever**.
HPI	Three weeks ago she was **scratched** on her right forearm **by her pet cat**; an erythematous pustule initially developed at the site but resolved spontaneously within 10 days.
PE	VS: fever. PE: **tender right axillary** and cervical **lymphadenopathy**.
Labs	Lymph node biopsy diagnostic; serologic indirect immunofluorescent antibody test for *Bartonella henselae* is positive.
Imaging	N/A
Gross Pathology	N/A
Micro Pathology	Hematoxylin and eosin staining reveals **granulomatous pathology** with stellate necrosis and surrounding palisades of histiocytic cells; **Warthin–Starry silver stain** reveals **clumps of pleomorphic, strongly argyrophilic bacilli**.
Treatment	Symptomatic; fluctuant node may need aspiration; antibiotics in immunosuppressed patients or those with severe disease.
Discussion	The cause of cat-scratch disease has yet to be clearly defined, but multiple organisms may be involved; *B. henselae* may be a more frequent cause of classic cat-scratch disease.

· ·

CAT-SCRATCH DISEASE

ID/CC	A 35-year-old male complains of **cough** productive of mucopurulent sputum and **breathlessness.**
HPI	Before the onset of these symptoms, he had a sore throat with hoarseness. He has no history of hemoptysis, sharp chest pain, or high-grade fever
PE	Creptitations heard over left lung base.
Labs	CBC: normal leukocyte count. Sputum exam revealed no **bacterial organism;** microimmunofluorescence detected species-specific antibodies directed against *Chlamydia* outer-membrane proteins; cultivation of *C. pneumoniae* demonstrated on HEp-2 and HL cell lines.
Imaging	CXR: left lower lobe subsegmental infiltrate with interstitial pattern.
Gross Pathology	N/A
Micro Pathology	N/A
Treatment	Tetracycline, doxycycline, or erythromycin.
Discussion	Overall, *Chlamydia pneumoniae* is responsible for approximately 6%–10% of all cases of pneumonia in the United States.

ID/CC	A 28-year-old male who lives in the **northwestern United States** complains of a high-grade **fever with rigors,** generalized aches, myalgias, headache, and backache.
HPI	Four days ago he returned from a hiking trip during which he was **bitten by a tick;** he took amoxicillin as prophylaxis against Lyme disease.
PE	VS: fever.
Labs	CBC: leukopenia; relative lymphocytosis. Viral antigen detected in RBCs by immunofluorescence; **Colorado tick virus cultured** in suckling mice by intracerebral inoculation of blood clot; indirect fluorescent Ab test positive.
Imaging	N/A
Gross Pathology	N/A
Micro Pathology	N/A
Treatment	Symptomatic.
Discussion	Colorado tick fever virus is an 80-nm double-shelled **reovirus** that is covered with capsomeres; its icosahedral core contains **12 segments of dsRNA.** The disease is a zoonosis that involves **hard (ixodid) ticks,** principally *Dermacentor andersoni,* and is endemic in the western and northwestern parts of the U.S. as well as in British Columbia and Alberta, Canada.

ID/CC	A 35-year-old male who works as a UN health worker presents with a high-grade **fever** and massive **hematemesis**.
HPI	He recently returned from **Zaire**, where he worked in a **tick-infested forest**.
PE	VS: fever. PE: extensive ecchymosis.
Labs	CBC: leukopenia; **severe thrombocytopenia. Crimean-Congo virus isolated.**
Imaging	N/A
Gross Pathology	N/A
Micro Pathology	N/A
Treatment	Supportive; **platelet transfusions; avoid salicylates;** barrier nursing and containment of infected secretions, since airborne infection may occur in hospital environment
Discussion	The agent responsible for Crimean-Congo hemorrhagic fever is a **bunyavirus; reservoirs** include wild and domesticated **sheep, cattle, goats, and hares.** The disease is transmitted by a **tick vector, usually an ixodid** of the genus *Hyalomma;* endemic areas include eastern Europe, Africa, Asia, Asia Minor, and the Indian subcontinent.

ID/CC	A **2-year-old** male is brought to the ER by his parents with **sore throat, inspiratory stridor,** and a barking cough of one day's duration.
HPI	The patient has no significant past medical history.
PE	VS: fever (38.6 C); tachypnea. PE: **respiratory distress;** nasopharyngeal discharge; diffuse rhonchi and wheezes; examination of extremities reveals some cyanosis.
Labs	Throat and nasal swabs isolate **parainfluenza virus;** serodiagnosis and hemagglutinin inhibition tests reveal type 2.
Imaging	CXR: air trapping. XR- Neck: **subglottic narrowing.**
Gross Pathology	Inflammation and edema of larynx, trachea, and bronchi.
Micro Pathology	N/A.
Treatment	Most cases respond to **supportive therapy** such as humidified air, removal of secretions, and bed rest. Severe cases may respond to **ribavirin** or high-dose **corticosteroids.**
Discussion	Differentiate from *H. influenzae* type B and influenza A virus. Spread by respiratory droplets; tends to peak in the fall or winter. Twenty percent of croup cases are caused by parainfluenza virus type 1.

. . . .

CROUP

ID/CC   A 10-year-old male is brought to the ER in a state of **shock** accompanied by **massive hematemesis.**

HPI   The family had just returned from a vacation in **Thailand.** His parents say that he had a high-grade fever for 5–6 days, for which he was receiving presumptive treatment for malaria.

PE   VS: hypotension; tachycardia. VS: cool, clammy extremities; **petechial skin rash** over extremities, axillae, trunk, and face; bleeding from venipuncture sites.

Labs   CBC: **thrombocytopenia; hematocrit increased** by > 20%. Abnormal clotting profile suggestive of **disseminated intravascular coagulation (DIC);** paired sera reveal significant rise in titer of hemagglutination inhibition antibodies against **Dengue virus serotypes 1 and 2.**

Imaging   US: bilateral pleural effusion and ascites.

Gross Pathology   N/A

Micro Pathology   N/A

Treatment   Symptomatic; manage shock; fresh blood/platelet-rich plasma; avoid salicylates.

Discussion   The disease is caused by a **mosquito-borne** (*Aedes aegypti*) **flavivirus** and is characterized by four distinct dengue serotypes. *A. aegypti* has a domestic habitat (stagnant water in flower pots, old jars, tin cans, and old tires) and bites during the day. Dengue fever is the principal endemo-epidemic disease entity in **Southeast Asia** (annual outbreaks occur in Burma, Thailand, Indonesia, and Vietnam) and has also been responsible for recent outbreaks in Cuba, other Caribbean islands, Venezuela, and Brazil. **FIRST AID** p.198

· ·

DENGUE HEMORRHAGIC FEVER

ID/CC   A 58-year-old man who was hitchhiking through **central and southern Africa** was admitted to a hospital in Zaire in a state of shock following **massive hemorrhage from the GI tract** (hematemesis and melena); he died within six hours of admission. Ten days later, a male **doctor who had attended** this patient and had attempted resuscitation became **ill with a similar disease** syndrome.

HPI   At admission, he gave an eight-day history of progressive **fever, myalgias, and watery diarrhea.** He also reported an erythematous, **measles-like skin rash** that had begun to desquamate.

PE   N/A

Labs   CBC: leukopenia; Pelger–Huët anomaly of neutrophils with atypical mononuclear cells; **thrombocytopenia with abnormal platelet aggregation.** Markedly elevated AST and ALT; blood was inoculated intraperitoneally into young guinea pigs and into various tissue culture cell lines, and **Ebola virus was detected by indirect immunofluorescent staining** techniques.

Imaging   N/A

Gross Pathology   At autopsy, **lymph nodes, liver, and spleen** found to be most conspicuously involved; stomach and intestines filled with blood; petechiae seen over bowel mucosa.

Micro Pathology   Severe congestion and stasis of spleen; **widespread necrosis of liver** cells; **electron microscopy** of liver revealed **pleomorphic virus particles** appearing in contrast preparations as **long, filamentous forms, U-shaped forms, and some circular forms resembling a doughnut.**

Treatment   **Outbreak was brought under control by** isolating patients, instituting **strict barrier nursing,** and **treatment of patient's excreta with disinfectants** such as formaldehyde and hypochlorite.

Discussion   A hemorrhagic, febrile infection of humans due to infection with the Ebola and Marburg viruses, both of which are filoviruses that are structurally indistinguishable but antigenically distinct. There is strong suspicion that this disease is a zoonosis, with monkeys initially being implicated. **FIRST AID** p.198

. . . .

EBOLA VIRUS HEMORRHAGIC FEVER

ID/CC	A 28-year-old male who is a resident of the **southeastern United States** presents with a high **fever with chills, headache, and myalgias.**
HPI	He remembers being **bitten by a tick** a week before developing his symptoms; however, he reports no skin rash.
PE	VS: fever. PE: no skin rash noted.
Labs	CBC: leukopenia and mild thrombocytopenia. **Characteristic intraleukocytic inclusion bodies** and serologic response to *Ehrlichia* antigens demonstrated; *E. chaffeensis* cultured from blood and detected by PCR.
Imaging	N/A
Gross Pathology	N/A
Micro Pathology	N/A
Treatment	Tetracycline.
Discussion	The agent of human ehrlichiosis has been attributed to a new *Ehrlichia* species, *E. chaffeensis,* which is most closely related to *E. canis. Ehrlichia* species are intraleukocytic parasites that are also pathogenic for a wide variety of wild and domestic animals.

EHRLICHIOSIS

ID/CC	A 30-year-old male from **Texas** presents with **fever and a skin rash** that began about two weeks ago.
HPI	The onset was gradual, with prodromal symptoms of headache, malaise, backache, and chills. These symptoms were followed by shaking chills, fever, and a more severe headache accompanied by nausea and vomiting. A remittent pattern of fever accompanied by tachycardia continued for 10–12 days, with the **rash appearing around the fifth day of fever.** The patient **worked at a rat-infested food-storage depot** this summer.
PE	VS: fever. PE: discrete, irregular pink **maculopapular rash** seen in axillae and on trunk, thighs, and upper arms; face, palms, and soles only sparsely involved; mild splenomegaly noted.
Labs	The **Weil–Felix** agglutination reaction for *Proteus* strain **OX-19 was positive;** complement-fixing antibodies to the typhus group antigen were demonstrated; **endemic typhus** (due to *Rickettsia typhi*) **was confirmed serologically** by using specific washed rickettsial antigens in IFA tests.
Imaging	N/A
Gross Pathology	N/A
Micro Pathology	N/A
Treatment	Antibiotic treatment with **chloramphenicol, tetracycline, or doxycycline.**
Discussion	Murine typhus is a natural infection of rats and mice by *Rickettsia typhi;* **spread of infection to humans by the rat flea** is incidental. The disease consists of fever, headache, myalgias, and a maculopapular rash.

ENDEMIC TYPHUS

ID/CC	A **3-day-old** female neonate presents with a **thick eye discharge.**
HPI	The **mother** admits to having **multiple sexual partners** and complains of a **vaginal discharge.** She did not receive adequate antenatal care.
PE	Exam of both eyes reveals a **thick purulent discharge** and marked **conjunctival congestion** and edema; conjunctival **chemosis** is so marked that cornea is seen at bottom of a crater-like pit; **corneal ulceration** noted.
Labs	Conjunctival swabs on Gram staining reveal presence of **gram-negative diplococci** both intra- and extracellularly in addition to **many PMNs;** conjunctival swab and maternal cervical culture yield *Neisseria gonorrhoeae.*
Imaging	N/A
Gross Pathology	N/A
Micro Pathology	N/A
Treatment	**Penicillin,** both topically and systemically; **cephalosporins (ceftriaxone)** for penicillinase-producing *N. gonorrhoeae.*
Discussion	Caused by *Neisseria gonorrhoeae,* the disease is **contracted** from a mother with gonorrhea **as the fetus passes down the birth canal;** infection does not occur in utero. **Corneal inflammation** is the major clinical sign that may produce complications like corneal opacities, perforation, anterior synechiae, anterior staphyloma, and panophthalmitis. It is now common practice to **prevent** this disease by treating the **eyes of the newborn with an antibacterial** compound; however, home childbirth bypasses this prophylactic procedure, and thus some cases are still occurring in the United States.

. . . .

GONOCOCCAL OPHTHALMIA NEONATORUM

ID/CC	A 56-year-old hospitalized male is found to have an abrupt-onset **high-grade fever** with chills a few hours after he underwent nephrolithotomy.
HPI	He was diagnosed with chronic nephrolithiasis with **recurrent UTIs**; a surgery intern also noted **poor urine output**.
PE	VS: fever; tachycardia; **hypotension**; tachypnea. VS: confused and disoriented; hyperventilating; diaphoresis; **hands warm** and pink with rapid capillary refill; pulse bounding; on chest auscultation, air entry found to be bilaterally reduced.
Labs	CBC: **leukocytosis** with left shift; neutrophils contain **toxic granulations, Döhle bodies,** and cytoplasmic vacuoles; band forms > 10%; thrombocytopenia. Prolongation of thrombin time, decreased fibrinogen, and presence of D-dimers (suggesting DIC); raised BUN and creatinine. ABGs: metabolic acidosis (increased anion gap due to lactic acidosis) and hypoxemia (due to **ARDS**). Blood and urine **culture yields** *E. coli.*
Imaging	CXR: evidence of noncardiogenic pulmonary edema (ARDS).
Gross Pathology	N/A
Micro Pathology	N/A
Treatment	**IV antibiotics** (with adequate gram-negative coverage); management of multiorgan failure (azotemia, ARDS, and DIC).
Discussion	Almost any bacterium can cause a bacteremia, including *E. coli* (most common), *Klebsiella, Proteus, Pseudomonas* (associated with antibiotic therapy and burn wounds), *Bacteroides fragilis* (causes of anaerobic septicemias), *S. aureus; S. pneumoniae,* and pediatric septicemia due to *E. coli* and *S. agalactiae.* Gram-negative bacteria release endotoxins; the release of endotoxin into the circulation leads to the activation of macrophages and monocytes, which in turn release cytokines. These cytokines trigger cascade reactions that lead to the clinical and biochemical manifestations of the sepsis syndrome.

· ·

GRAM-NEGATIVE SEPSIS

ID/CC	A 28-year-old male **immigrant** presents with **inguinal swelling** and a **painless penile ulcer.**
HPI	He admits to unprotected intercourse with **multiple sexual partners,** many of whom were prostitutes.
PE	Soft, **painless,** raised, **raw, beef-colored,** smooth **granulating ulcer** noted on distal penis; multiple **subcutaneous swellings** (= PSEUDOBUBOES) noted in inguinal region, some of which have ulcerated.
Labs	Giemsa-stained smear from penile and inguinal regions demonstrate characteristic "**closed safety pin**" appearance of encapsulated organisms **within a large histiocyte** (= DONOVAN BODIES).
Imaging	N/A
Gross Pathology	N/A
Micro Pathology	Characteristic histologic picture of donovanosis comprises some degree of epithelial hyperplasia at margins of lesions; dense plasma cell infiltrate scatters histiocyte-containing Donovan bodies.
Treatment	Tetracycline; cotrimoxazole.
Discussion	Granuloma inguinale, a slowly progressive, ulcerative, granulomatous STD involving the genitalia, is caused by the gram-negative bacillus *Calymmatobacterium granulomatis* (formerly *Donovania granulomatis*); it is seen in Giemsa-stained sections as a dark-staining, encapsulated, intracellular rod-shaped inclusion in macrophages, the so-called **Donovan body.**

GRANULOMA INGUINALE

ID/CC	A **60-year-old male** presents with **cough productive of mucopurulent sputum** together with mild fever and worsening breathlessness.
HPI	He is a chronic smoker who has been diagnosed with **COPD**.
PE	VS: fever. PE: in moderate respiratory distress; emphysematous chest with obliterated cardiac and liver dullness; **wheezing and crepts** heard over both lung fields
Labs	*H. influenzae* organisms seen as small, pleomorphic gram-negative bacilli on Gram stain of sputum; **nontypable *H. influenzae* isolated on sputum culture** (to grow in culture, *H. influenzae* requires both factor X–hematin and factor V–nicotinamide nucleoside present in erythrocytes).
Imaging	N/A
Gross Pathology	N/A
Micro Pathology	N/A
Treatment	**Amoxicillin/ampicillin therapy;** SMX–TMP, ciprofloxacin, ofloxacin, and clarithromycin are also excellent drugs for the treatment of clinically mild to moderate *H. influenzae* infections of the upper respiratory tract.
Discussion	Infections caused by nontypable, or unencapsulated, *H. influenzae* strains have been increasingly recognized in pediatric and adult populations. Nontypable *H. influenzae* strains are frequent respiratory tract colonizers in patients with COPD and commonly exacerbate chronic bronchitis in these patients; nontypable strains are also the most common cause of acute otitis media in children. **FIRST AID** p.183

· ·

H. INFLUENZAE UPPER RESPIRATORY TRACT INFECTION

ID/CC	A 25-year-old male presented with sudden-onset **breathlessness, cough, cyanosis, and high-grade fever.**
HPI	The patient failed to improve on 100% oxygen, became hypotensive, and **died of type 2 respiratory failure** a few hours after admission. He had been in perfect health and had been **hiking in several rodent-infested areas** before falling ill.
PE	On admission he was found to have fever, tachycardia, **cyanosis,** hypotension, and **rales on auscultation** over both lung fields; no meningeal signs or localizing CNS signs could be demonstrated.
Labs	ABGs: respiratory acidosis with **hypoxia and hypercapnia.** CBC: leukocytosis; **hemoconcentration; thrombocytopenia;** atypical lymphocytosis. Increased LDH and ALT levels; prolonged PT index; sputum exam and blood culture did not yield any organism; IgM antibody to hantavirus and immunohistochemical stains for **hantavirus antigen in tissues confirmed** infection with the virus.
Imaging	CXR: **noncardiogenic pulmonary edema** (bat-wing edema pattern).
Gross Pathology	N/A
Micro Pathology	Histopathologic exam of lung tissues was suggestive of **acute respiratory distress syndrome** (adult hyaline membrane disease).
Treatment	Patient died despite **intensive ventilatory support.**
Discussion	A virus closely related to the **Hantaan virus** (which produces Korean hemorrhagic fever and hemorrhagic fever with renal syndrome) has been recovered from mice in various regions of the United States; **rodents are the natural host** for this group of viruses. Infected rodents shed the virus in saliva, urine, and feces for many weeks, and **humans** are believed to **acquire the infection via exposure to rodent excrement or saliva,** either by the aerosol route or by direct inoculation. **FIRST AID** p.198

HANTAVIRUS PULMONARY SYNDROME

ID/CC	A 25-year-old male woodcutter, residing in **S. Korea,** is admitted to the ER in a state of **shock and massive epistaxis.**
HPI	The patient had been complaining of fever, malaise, headache, myalgias, back pain, abdominal pain, nausea, and vomiting for the past week; he also complained of **extremely reduced urine output.** Careful history revealed that before he fell ill, he and his friend were cutting wood in the forest when they accidentally **disturbed a rodent-infested area.**
PE	VS: hypotension. PE: **epistaxis;** facial flushing; petechiae and subconjunctival hemorrhages.
Labs	Deranged RFTs suggestive of **acute renal failure.** CBC: **thrombocytopenia.** Serology and **culture identify hantavirus, Hantaan serotype.**
Imaging	N/A
Gross Pathology	N/A
Micro Pathology	N/A
Treatment	Supportive management in the form of dialysis (**for renal failure**); management of shock and hemorrhage; **IV ribavirin.**
Discussion	Korean hemorrhagic fever with renal syndrome is caused by **the Hantaan serotype of hantavirus.** Its **reservoirs are various rodents found in diverse areas** of the world, and the **infection spreads directly** from an animal reservoir to humans without transmission by a vector.

. . . .

HEMORRHAGIC FEVER RENAL SYNDROME

ID/CC	A 7-year-old male complains of a **high fever** and a very **sore throat.**
HPI	The pain is so severe that the child refuses to swallow. He is adequately immunized and achieved normal developmental milestones.
PE	VS: fever. PE: **characteristic vesicular lesions** scattered over **soft palate, tonsils, and pharynx.**
Labs	Coxsackievirus A isolated from mucosal lesions.
Imaging	N/A
Gross Pathology	N/A
Micro Pathology	N/A
Treatment	Self-limiting condition.
Discussion	In **hand, foot, and mouth disease** (HFMD), in addition to the oral lesions, there are similar lesions seen over the palms, soles, and buttocks. Herpangina may be caused by coxsackievirus A1 through A10, A16, and A22; outbreaks of HFMD are usually caused by coxsackievirus A16.

HERPANGINA

ID/CC	A 60-year-old male presents with **swelling and a vesicular skin eruption on the left side of his face.**
HPI	The patient reports that before the rash developed, he had severe radiating pain on the left side of his face. He also recalls having suffered an attack of **chickenpox during his childhood.**
PE	**Unilateral vesicular rash** accompanied in places by suppuration, bleeding, and small pitted scars over left forehead, nasal bridge, including tip (indicating involvement of the **nasociliary branch** of the trigeminal nerve), left side of nose, and periorbital area; skin of lids red and edematous; slit-lamp examination reveals numerous rounded spots composed of minute white dots involving epithelium and stroma, producing a **coarse subepithelial punctate keratitis; cornea** is **insensitive.**
Labs	N/A
Imaging	N/A
Gross Pathology	N/A
Micro Pathology	Vesicular skin lesions with **herpesvirus inclusions** that are **intranuclear and acidophilic** with a clear halo around them (**Cowdry type A inclusion bodies**); syncytial giant cells also seen.
Treatment	Acyclovir; steroids.
Discussion	Caused by the **varicella zoster virus,** which causes chickenpox as a primary infection. Zoster is believed to be a **reactivation of the latent viral infection.** In **zoster ophthalmicus,** the chief **focus of reactivation is the trigeminal ganglion,** from which the virus travels down one or more branches of the ophthalmic division such that its area of distribution is marked out by rows of vesicles or scars left by the vesicles. **Ocular complications** arise during subsidence of the rash and are generally **associated with** involvement of the **nasociliary branch** of the trigeminal nerve.

HERPES ZOSTER OPHTHALMICUS

ID/CC   An 18-year-old male complains of severe **irritation** in the left eye, excessive **lacrimation, and photophobia.**

HPI   He reports that he has had **similar episodes** in the past that were treated with an antiviral drug. His records indicate that he suffered the **first attack** at the age of seven, at which time his condition was diagnosed and treated **as a severe follicular keratoconjunctivitis;** his records also indicate a history of **recurrent** episodes of **herpes labialis.**

PE   Examination of left eye reveals circumcorneal congestion; fluorescein staining of cornea reveals infiltrates spreading in all directions, coalescing with each other and forming a **large, shallow ulcer with crenated edges** (= "DENDRITIC ULCER"); cornea is **insensitive.**

Labs   HSV-1 demonstrated on immunofluorescent staining of epithelial scrapings as well as in the aqueous humor.

Imaging   N/A

Gross Pathology   N/A

Micro Pathology   N/A

Treatment   **Trifluorothymidine and acyclovir are effective; steroids are contraindicated.**

Discussion   Most ocular herpetic infections are **caused by HSV-1.** Primary infections present as unilateral follicular conjunctivitis, blepharitis, or corneal epithelial opacities; **recurrences** may take the **form of keratitis** (> 90% of cases are unilateral), blepharitis, or keratoconjunctivitis. **Branching dendritic ulcers,** usually detected by fluorescein staining, are virtually diagnostic; deep stromal involvement may result in scarring, corneal thinning, and abnormal vascularization with resulting blindness or rupture of the globe.

. . . .

HSV KERATITIS

ID/CC	A **2-day-old** neonate is evaluated for an **eye discharge**.
HPI	The baby's **mother is a prostitute** who did not receive any prenatal cervical cultures during pregnancy.
PE	Normal full-term male neonate; mucoid **eye discharge, conjunctival congestion, and chemosis** noted in both eyes; nonfollicles seen on palpebral conjunctiva (due to absence of subconjunctival adenoid layer at this age); mild **superficial keratitis** also present.
Labs	Gram stain of swab reveals increased **PMNs** and **no bacteria**; characteristic **intracellular inclusion bodies demonstrated by the DIF test**; cell culture yields *Chlamydia trachomatis* **serotypes D–K**; chlamydia also grown from **maternal cervical swab**.
Imaging	N/A
Gross Pathology	N/A
Micro Pathology	N/A
Treatment	**Erythromycin** systemically; **chlortetracycline** ointment topically.
Discussion	*Chlamydia trachomatis* strains can be further differentiated into 18 serotypes by microimmunofluorescence tests. **Serotypes A, B, Ba, and C** are principally associated with **endemic trachoma** in developing countries; **serotypes D–K** primarily cause **sexually transmitted** infections in adults and **inclusion conjunctivitis and pneumonia in infants**, transmitted through an infected birth canal; **serotypes L1, L2, and L3** cause **lymphogranuloma venereum**.

· ·

INCLUSION CONJUNCTIVITIS

ID/CC	A 65-year-old male presents with a **high fever,** headache, extreme prostration, a **nonproductive cough,** and severe **breathlessness.**
HPI	He had been receiving chlorambucil for treatment of chronic lymphocytic leukemia (CLL) and was in an extremely **debilitated state.**
PE	VS: fever; tachypnea; cyanosis. PE: **conjunctival congestion; pharyngeal inflammation; rales** heard on auscultation over both lung fields; splenomegaly and lymphadenopathy (due to CLL).
Labs	No organisms seen or cultured from sputum; fluorescent antibody directed against **influenza virus** was positive; viral cultures of nasopharyngeal washings grew influenza virus; fourfold rise in **hemagglutination inhibition antibody titer** against influenza virus demonstrated.
Imaging	CXR (PA view): bilateral, diffuse interstitial infiltrates suggestive of **atypical pneumonia.**
Gross Pathology	N/A
Micro Pathology	N/A
Treatment	**Amantidine;** ventilatory support, antipyretics, and IV fluids. Development of **secondary staphylococcal pneumonia** should be treated with parenteral antibiotics; **yearly vaccination** prevents excessive morbidity and mortality, especially among the elderly.
Discussion	Influenza viruses are medium-sized spherical **RNA viruses termed orthomyxoviruses;** influenza A and B viruses each contain 8 RNA segments and 10 viral proteins. Influenza infection is **most common in winter,** with the **severity** of a given influenza **outbreak depending on the status of immunity** in the community. Previous natural infection or immunization with viruses that are immunologically close to the current strain limits new infection; however, if **antigenic drift** results in reduced cross-reactivity, the new strain will spread more rapidly. New strains produced by **antigenic shift** account for most major outbreaks. Influenza affects all segments of the population, but severe infections and **major complications** are most common **in patients who are young,** elderly, or debilitated. **FIRST AID** p.198

INFLUENZA

ID/CC	A 30-year-old female presents with **fever, chills,** malaise, headaches, and **myalgias.**
HPI	She was diagnosed as suffering from **secondary syphilis** with an extensive nonpruritic **skin rash, condylomata lata,** and **mucous patches** in the mouth, for which she received a dose of intramuscular **penicillin six hours ago.**
PE	VS: **fever;** tachycardia; mild hypotension.
Labs	N/A
Imaging	N/A
Gross Pathology	N/A
Micro Pathology	N/A
Treatment	No specific treatment; symptoms subside in 24 hours.
Discussion	The Jarisch–Herxheimer reaction consists of fever, chills, mild hypotension, headache, and an increase in the intensity of mucocutaneous lesions **6–8 hours after** initiating **treatment of syphilis with penicillin** or another effective antibiotic; symptoms usually **subside in 12–24 hours.** The reaction has been reported in 50% of patients with primary syphilis and in 75% of those with secondary syphilis. The Jarisch–Herxheimer reaction **also occurs after treatment of other spirochetal diseases** (e.g., louse-borne relapsing fever caused by *Borrelia recurrentis*). It has been suggested that the release of treponemal lipopolysaccharides might produce this symptom complex.

. . . .

JARISCH–HERXHEIMER REACTION

ID/CC   A 4-year-old Japanese male presents with complaints of **fever and an extensive skin rash.**

HPI   He had previously been diagnosed with cervical adenitis by a primary care physician, who administered antibiotics to no effect.

PE   VS: fever. PE: **conjunctival congestion;** dry, red lips; erythematous palms and soles; indurative edema of the peripheral extremities; **desquamation of fingertips; rash on trunk; cervical lymphadenopathy.**

Labs   Throat swab and culture sterile. CBC: routine blood counts normal; further differential blood counts revealed increased B-cell activation and T-helper cell lymphocytopenia. Paul–Bunnell test for infectious mononucleosis was negative; serologic tests ruled out CMV infection and toxoplasmosis.

Imaging   Angio: **presence of coronary artery aneurysms.**

Gross Pathology   N/A

Micro Pathology   **Coronary arteritis** is usually demonstrated at autopsy together with aneurysm formation and thrombosis. **Fatalities in this syndrome are due primarily to coronary insufficiency.**

Treatment   **Aspirin and intravenous gamma globulin** are effective in preventing coronary complications if initiated early.

Discussion   The disease is usually self-limited, but in a few instances **fatal coronary thrombosis** has occurred during the acute stage of the disease or many months after apparently complete recovery. Case-fatality rates have been about 1%–2%. The etiology of this disease is unknown.

KAWASAKI SYNDROME

ID/CC	A 30-year-old male from **India** presents with slowly progressive **hypopigmented skin patches and nodules** together with a peculiar **deformity of the nose.**
HPI	The patient has a history of **nasal stuffiness** and bloody nasal discharge; he also complains of **loss of libido.**
PE	**Leonine facies;** loss of eyebrows (= MADAROSIS); scleral nodules; **depressed nasal bridge** (= "SADDLE-NOSE" DEFORMITY); gynecomastia; **testicular atrophy;** numerous **symmetrical, hypopigmented macules with vague edges** and erythematous, smooth, shiny surfaces; skin plaques and nodules; **partial loss of pinprick and temperature sensation** (= HYPOESTHESIA); no anhidrotic changes; symmetrically **enlarged ulnar and common peroneal nerves.**
Labs	Slit skin smears: **numerous acid-fast bacilli** on modified ZN staining.
Imaging	N/A
Gross Pathology	N/A
Micro Pathology	Dermis massively and diffusely infiltrated with **foamy histiocytes with bacilli and globi** (masses of acid-fast bacilli) containing Virchow giant cells; bacilli found only rarely in epidermis and in subepidermal "**clear zone**"; epidermis thinned out with flattening of rete ridges.
Treatment	Multidrug therapy with **rifampicin, dapsone, clofazimine.**
Discussion	The discovery of one or more of the following is pathognomonic of leprosy: (1) **anesthetic skin lesions** (found in all tuberculoid and many lepromatous cases); (2) **thickening of one or more nerves** (found in many lepromatous and some tuberculoid cases); and (3) the presence of **acid-fast bacilli in skin smears** (found in all lepromatous and some tuberculoid cases). *Mycobacterium leprae* has not been cultured in vitro thus far. **FIRST AID** p.185

LEPROMATOUS LEPROSY

ID/CC
A 35-year-old British **dairy farmer** complains of a high remittent **fever** with chills, severe muscle aches, **decreased urine output,** and **dark-colored urine** for the past two days.

HPI
He also complains of an extensive skin rash and nasal bleeding (= EPISTAXIS). A careful history reveals that the area in which he works is infested with rodents.

PE
VS: **fever;** tachycardia; hypotension. PE: **icterus;** extensive hemorrhagic maculopapular skin eruption; **conjunctival suffusion;** lymphadenopathy.

Labs
CBC: leukocytosis with neutrophilia. Mild **hyperbilirubinemia,** predominantly conjugated; **increased alkaline phosphatase; elevated BUN and creatinine.** UA: proteinuria, **casts,** and RBCs. Blood culture (positive during first 10 days of illness) and urine culture (positive after second week of infection) on Fletcher's medium isolated *Leptospira interrogans;* serologic diagnosis (positive during second week of illness): microscopic slide agglutination demonstrated significant titer of antibody to *L. interrogans.*

Imaging
N/A

Gross Pathology
Severe infection damages both the **liver and kidneys.**

Micro Pathology
Liver biopsy shows focal centrilobular necrosis with focal lymphocytic infiltration and disorganization of liver cell plates together with proliferation of Kupffer cells with cholestasis; kidney biopsy reveals mesangial proliferation with PMN infiltration; electron microscopy reveals dense deposits in basement membrane and subepithelial area.

Treatment
Penicillin (dose modified due to presence of renal failure), doxycycline; hemodialysis.

Discussion
Weil's disease, a severe form of leptospirosis caused by *Leptospira interrogans* complex, is characterized by fever, jaundice, cutaneous and visceral hemorrhages, anemia, azotemia, and altered consciousness; major vectors to humans are rodents. Transmission occurs through direct contact with the blood, tissue, or urine of infected animals.

· ·

LEPTOSPIROSIS

ID/CC	A **6-year-old male** is brought to the ER in a **delirious state** with fever and marked **dyspnea** that have rapidly progressed over the past two days.
HPI	His **mother,** an **Asian immigrant,** was diagnosed and treated for **pulmonary tuberculosis** a few months ago. He has had a low-grade **fever,** cough, **malaise,** and **night sweats** for the past two months. The child has not received prophylactic isoniazid or BCG vaccination.
PE	VS: fever; tachycardia; marked tachypnea; hypotension. PE: toxic and stuporous; pallor; **central cyanosis;** extensive rales and rhonchi bilaterally; hepatosplenomegaly; funduscopy reveals **choroidal tubercles.**
Labs	CBC: **lymphocytosis;** normochromic, normocytic anemia. **Increased ESR; Mantoux skin test negative;** staining and culture of transbronchial and bone marrow biopsy specimens reveal presence of *Mycobacterium tuberculosis;* PCR for tuberculosis positive; ELISA for HIV negative.
Imaging	CXR: soft, **uniformly distributed fine nodules throughout both lung fields** (= MILIARY MOTTLING).
Gross Pathology	Myriad 1- to 2-mm **granulomas** demonstrable in lungs, liver, and bone marrow biopsy specimens.
Micro Pathology	**Granulomas** with **central caseous necrosis** surrounded by epithelial cells, Langhans cells, lymphocytes, plasma cells, and fibroblasts in affected tissues.
Treatment	**Multidrug antitubercular therapy** with isoniazid, rifampicin, pyrazinamide, and ethambutol or streptomycin; steroids may be indicated.
Discussion	Miliary tuberculosis results from **widespread hematogenous dissemination** and often presents with a perplexing fever, dyspnea, anemia, and splenomegaly; the disease is **more fulminant in children** than in adults. **FIRST AID** p.185

ID/CC	A 50-year-old diabetic male presents with **fever, pain, and a necrotizing swelling** over his left leg.
HPI	His symptoms began about a week ago with redness and swelling of the left leg followed by bronze discoloration of the skin and the appearance of hemorrhagic bullae.
PE	Extensive cutaneous **gangrene** observed over left leg with many ruptured bullae; black necrotic eschar with surrounding erythema resembles a third-degree burn.
Labs	Swab staining reveals presence of chains of gram-positive cocci; culture isolated **beta-hemolytic group A streptococcus** (*S. pyogenes*).
Imaging	N/A
Gross Pathology	N/A
Micro Pathology	Biopsy specimen reveals areas of necrosis in dermis and subcutaneous fat, infiltration with PMNs, and vasculitis and thrombosis in vessels in the superficial fascia.
Treatment	**Removal of necrotic fascia in conjunction with high-dose penicillin.**
Discussion	Streptococcal gangrene is a group A streptococcal cellulitis that rapidly progresses to gangrene of the subcutaneous tissue and necrosis of the overlying skin; the disease process usually involves an extremity. Necrotizing fasciitis is now recognized as the consequence of mixed bacterial infections caused by anaerobes, facultative gram-negative bacilli, and enterococci. The term "synergistic necrotizing cellulitis" applies to this type of polymicrobic necrotizing fasciitis.

NECROTIZING FASCIITIS

ID/CC	A 60-year-old male who was hospitalized following a stroke presents with a high-grade **fever with chills** and obtundation.
HPI	He had been **catheterized due to urinary incontinence and was receiving cephalosporin** for treatment of aspiration pneumonitis.
PE	VS: fever.
Labs	**Blood culture** grew *Enterococcus faecalis* (morphologically indistinguishable from streptococci and immunologically similar to members of group D streptococci, the enterococci are metabolically unique in their ability to resist heat, bile, and 6.5% NaCl); urine culture also isolated *S. fecalis*.
Imaging	N/A
Gross Pathology	N/A
Micro Pathology	N/A
Treatment	**Ampicillin and gentamicin with vancomycin.**
Discussion	Enterococci constitute a relatively common cause of UTIs, wound infections, and peritonitis and intra-abdominal abscesses; enterococci have become an increasingly prominent cause of **bacteremia,** which usually originates from a **focus in the urinary tract or abdomen.** The incidence of nosocomial bacteremias caused by these organisms is also increasing, particularly in patients who have received cephalosporins or other broad-spectrum antibiotics. All clinically significant isolates should be subjected to testing for **beta-lactamase production,** high-level **aminoglycoside resistance,** and **vancomycin resistance** to determine if an alternative therapy is necessary. Infections caused by enterococci that produce beta-lactamase are treated with an antimicrobial agent that combines a penicillin with a beta-lactamase inhibitor; infections caused by strains that are highly resistant to aminoglycosides are treated with vancomycin.

. . . .

NOSOCOMIAL ENTEROCOCCAL INFECTION

ID/CC   A 20-year-old male swimmer complains of severe **pain** and **itching** in the right ear that is associated with a slight amount of **yellowish** (= PURULENT) **discharge.**

HPI   The patient has no previous history of discharge from the ear and no history of associated deafness or tinnitus.

PE   Red, swollen area seen in right external auditory meatus that is partially obliterating the lumen; **movement of tragus** is exquisitely **painful** (= TRAGAL SIGN).

Labs   Gram stain of aural swab reveals presence of gram negative rods; culture isolates *Pseudomonas aeruginosa.*

Imaging   N/A

Gross Pathology   Red, swollen area seen in cartilaginous part of external auditory meatus; when visualized, tympanic membrane is erythematous and moves normally with pneumatic otoscopy (vs. acute otitis media).

Micro Pathology   N/A

Treatment   Antibiotics; gentle removal of debris in ear.

Discussion   Most common in summer months and thought to arise from a change in the milieu of the external auditory meatus by increased alkalization and excessive moisture; this leads to bacterial overgrowth, most commonly with gram-negative rods like *Pseudomonas* (also causes malignant otitis externa) and *Proteus* or fungi like *Aspergillus.*

. . . .

OTITIS EXTERNA

ID/CC	A 9-year-old male is admitted for an evaluation of a **suspected** underlying **immune deficiency.**
HPI	He has been hospitalized and treated several times for **recurrent** life-threatening **septicemia due to** *S. pneumoniae,* **meningococcus,** and *H. influenzae.* Careful history reveals that a few years ago he underwent an emergency **splenectomy** following traumatic splenic rupture in a motor vehicle accident.
PE	Left paramedian postsurgical scar seen on abdomen.
Labs	Reduced IgM levels; **reduced antibody production when challenged with particulate antigens.**
Imaging	US-Abdomen: **spleen is absent.**
Gross Pathology	N/A
Micro Pathology	N/A
Treatment	**Pneumococcal vaccine and prophylactic antibiotics** (penicillin or erythromycin)
Discussion	Patients who have undergone **splenectomy or** who are **functionally asplenic** are at increased **risk for overwhelming bacteremia;** pathogens include **organisms that possess a polysaccharide capsule,** such as meningococcus, *Staphylococcus,* the DF2 bacillus, and, especially, *S. pneumoniae* and *H. influenzae* type B. Such **functionally asplenic** patients include individuals with **sickle cell disease** and those who have undergone **splenic irradiation. Pneumococcal vaccine** is indicated in all patients who have undergone splenectomy, particularly children and adolescents.

. . . .

OVERWHELMING POSTSPLENECTOMY SEPSIS

ID/CC   A 25-year-old HIV-negative **homosexual male** presents with rectal burning, itching in the anal region, **tenesmus,** and a **bloody, mucopurulent discharge** per rectum.

HPI   One month ago he was hospitalized with severe **febrile proctocolitis** that was diagnosed as **lymphogranuloma venereum.** He has also been treated several times in the past for amebiasis and shigella colitis and admits to having **receptive anal intercourse.** Further history reveals that his most recent **sexual partner** has been suffering from **urethral pain and discharge.**

PE   Condylomata acuminata noted in perianal distribution; remainder of physical exam normal.

Labs   Gram stain and culture of **rectal swab** reveals gram-negative diplococci identified as *Neisseria gonorrhoeae* on Thayer–Martin medium; urethral swab from partner also isolates *N. gonorrhoeae.*

Imaging   Sigmoidoscopy: proctitis with bloody mucopurulent discharge noted.

Gross Pathology   N/A

Micro Pathology   N/A

Treatment   **Ceftriaxone** and **doxycycline** (to treat likely concomitant Chlamydial infection) for both patient and partner. Most apparent failures of correct antibiotic therapy are in fact due to reinfection; in resistant cases, **spectinomycin** may be used.

Discussion   The term **"gay bowel syndrome"** is used in reference to enteric and perirectal infections that are commonly encountered in immune-competent homosexual men; in homosexuals with HIV, opportunistic organisms play a more important role. Common etiologic agents include *Chlamydia trachomatis,* lymphogranuloma venereum serovars, *N. gonorrhoeae,* HSV, *Treponema pallidum,* human papilloma virus, *Campylobacter* species, *Shigella, Entamoeba histolytica,* and *Giardia.*

PROCTOCOLITIS

ID/CC A 35-year-old male presents with high **fever,** malaise, headache, and a **hacking cough productive** of a small amount of mucoid sputum.

HPI He has two **pet parrots** at home who have recently shown **signs of illness.**

PE VS: fever; **bradycardia.** PE: auscultation of chest reveals **crepitant rales** over both lower lung fields; **splenomegaly** with mild hepatomegaly noted; multiple **purpuric macules** seen over abdomen (= "HORDER'S SPOTS").

Labs Greater than fourfold rise in complement-fixing antibody titer to a group antigen suggestive of infection with *Chlamydia psittaci;* definitive diagnosis of psittacosis was made from sputum by isolation of *C. psittaci* in pretreated tissue culture cells.

Imaging CXR-PA: **interstitial** patchy, bilateral **infiltrates.**

Gross Pathology Principal lesions found in lungs, liver and spleen.

Micro Pathology Pulmonary lesion is an **interstitial pneumonitis;** mononuclear cells with ballooned cytoplasm containing inclusion bodies are observed. In the liver, focal necrosis of hepatocyte occurs along with Kupffer cell hyperplasia.

Treatment **Tetracycline/doxycycline.**

Discussion Psittacosis is an acute infection caused by *Chlamydia psittaci;* it is characterized primarily by pneumonitis and systemic manifestations and is **transmitted** to humans by a variety of avian species, **principally psittacine birds (parrots, parakeets).** A history of contact with birds, particularly sick birds, or of employment in a pet shop or in the poultry industry provides a clue to the diagnosis of psittacosis in a patient with pneumonia, especially if bradycardia and splenomegaly are also present.

· ·

PSITTACOSIS

ID/CC	A 30-year-old **dairy farm worker** presents with complaints of **fever, cough, pleuritic chest pain,** and malaise.
HPI	His work at the dairy involves **milking cows** and **looking after parturient cattle.**
PE	VS: fever; tachypnea. PE: mild icterus; bilateral **crackles** on chest auscultation.
Labs	CBC: normal WBC count. Mild elevation of serum bilirubin and liver enzymes; greater than fourfold increase in **complement-fixing antibody (against *Coxiella burnetii*)** titer between acute and convalescent sera (IFA technique for early detection of specific IgM Ab is the serodiagnostic method of choice); **negative Weil–Felix reaction;** *C. burnetii* isolated from sputum by inoculation of cultured human fetal diploid fibroblasts.
Imaging	CXR: right upper lobe **rounded opacity** that increased in size over a few days and cleared completely with treatment.
Gross Pathology	N/A
Micro Pathology	N/A
Treatment	Tetracycline, doxycycline.
Discussion	Q fever is caused by the rickettsia-like organism *Coxiella burnetii* and produces the clinical picture of primary atypical pneumonia. Q fever differs from the other human rickettsioses in that rash is absent and **transmission** is usually **by the airborne route.** *C. burnetii* localizes in the **mammary glands and uterus of pregnant cattle,** sheep, and goats, in which infection is mild or inapparent; **infected placentas, postpartum discharges, and the feces of these animals** are the **principal sources of contaminated material** in the environment. Humans acquire Q fever by inhaling aerosolized particles from such substances; particularly **at risk** are **dairy and slaughterhouse workers.**

Q FEVER

ID/CC	A 27-year-old male **researcher** presents with sudden-onset **fever,** chills, headache, a **skin rash,** and **painful** swelling of multiple limb **joints.**
HPI	Careful history reveals that he was **bitten by a rat** in his laboratory a few days ago; the bite wound has now healed.
PE	VS: **fever.** PE: morbilliform **rash** noted over extremities, particularly the hands and feet; **painful swelling** and restriction of movement noted over **both wrist and knee joints.**
Labs	CBC: leukocytosis. *Streptobacillus moniliformis* isolated from blood and synovial fluid of inflamed joints; agglutinins to *S. moniliformis* demonstrated in significant titers.
Imaging	N/A
Gross Pathology	N/A
Micro Pathology	N/A
Treatment	**Penicillin.**
Discussion	Rat-bite fever, which is caused by *Streptococcus moniliformis,* is an acute febrile illness that is usually accompanied by a skin rash; **most cases result from the bites of wild or lab rats,** although mice, squirrels, weasels, dogs, and cats may also transmit the disease by bites or scratches. The disease is called **Haverhill fever** when *S. moniliformis* is transmitted by drinking rat-excrement-contaminated milk. Distribution is probably worldwide, with most cases occurring in crowded cities characterized by poor sanitation.

. . . .

RAT BITE FEVER

ID/CC	A 30-year-old male who lives in the **western part of the U.S.** presents with **high fever,** shaking **chills,** severe headache, myalgias, and diarrhea.
HPI	He reports having had **similar symptoms 10 days ago** that lasted for 4–5 days, followed by defervescence accompanied by drenching sweats and marked prostration. He had been **hiking in a tick-infested forest** until about a week before the development of symptoms.
PE	VS: **fever.**
Labs	**Spirochetes found on thick smears of peripheral blood** obtained during febrile period and **stained with Wright or Giemsa stain.**
Imaging	N/A
Gross Pathology	N/A
Micro Pathology	N/A
Treatment	**Tetracycline** is the drug of choice; chloramphenicol or penicillin may also be used.
Discussion	Relapsing fever is an **acute louse-borne or tick-borne infection** that is caused by blood spirochetes of the genus *Borrelia;* it is characterized by **recurrent febrile episodes separated by asymptomatic intervals.** Unlike other spirochetes, the etiologic agent can readily be detected with Giemsa stain or Wright's stain. *B. recurrentis* is the **cause of louse-borne relapsing fever,** whereas a variety of different species produce the **tick-borne disease.** In the United States, the predominant species are *B. hermsii* and *B. turicatae.*

· ·

RELAPSING FEVER

ID/CC	A **5-month-old** male infant is brought to the pediatric clinic with **wheezing and respiratory difficulty** of three hours' duration.
HPI	He has had rhinorrhea, fever, and cough and had been sneezing for two days prior to her visit to the clinic.
PE	VS: tachypnea. PE: nasal flaring; mild **central cyanosis**; accessory muscle use during respiration; hyperexpansion of chest; **expiratory and inspiratory wheezes; rhonchi** over both lung fields.
Labs	CBC/PBS: relative lymphocytosis. ABGs: hypoxemia with mild hypercapnia. Normal flora on bacterial culture of sputum; **respiratory syncytial virus (RSV)** demonstrated on viral culture of throat swab.
Imaging	CXR: hyperinflation; segmental atelectasis; interstitial infiltrates.
Gross Pathology	N/A
Micro Pathology	N/A
Treatment	Humidified oxygen; bronchodilators; aerosolized **ribavirin**.
Discussion	RSV is the **most common cause of bronchiolitis in infants** under two years of age; other viral causes include parainfluenza, influenza, and adenovirus. **FIRST AID** p.198

· ·

RSV PNEUMONIA

ID/CC	A 14-year-old male who is known to have **sickle cell anemia** presents with throbbing **pain, redness,** and **swelling** of the **right thigh.**
HPI	The patient also complains of fever and chills of one week's duration. He has a few **pet turtles** at home.
PE	VS: **fever**; tachycardia. PE: pallor; redness, swelling, and tenderness over right thigh; effusion demonstrated in right knee joint; limitation of range of motion of right knee.
Labs	CBC: leukocytosis; elevated ESR. PBS: irreversible **sickling;** blood culture reveals *Salmonella choleraesuis;* organism also isolated from pus aspirated from right femur (diagnostic of **osteomyelitis**).
Imaging	Nuc: **increased uptake in metaphyseal region** of right femur. XR: (usually normal during the first 10 days of illness) may reveal changes of bone resorption, detached necrotic cortical bone (= SEQUESTRUM) and laminated periosteal new-bone formation (= INVOLUCRUM).
Gross Pathology	Dense, pale, sclerotic-appearing area in shaft.
Micro Pathology	Changes range from suppurative and ischemic destructive necrosis, fibrosis, and ultimate bone repair.
Treatment	**Parenteral antibiotics** (chloramphenicol, fluoroquinolones, third-generation cephalosporins); **surgical** drainage of abscess, sequestra removal, and necrotic bone resection.
Discussion	A striking association has been noted between diseases producing hemolysis (e.g., sickle cell anemia, malaria, and bartonellosis) and *Salmonella* infections; elderly patients with impaired host defense mechanisms, those with hepatosplenic schistosomiasis, and AIDS patients are also at increased risk of severe and recurrent *Salmonella* bacteremia.

· ·

SALMONELLA SEPTICEMIA WITH OSTEOMYELITIS

ID/CC	An Asian refugee **family** comprising a 30-year-old man, his wife, and two schoolchildren present **with complaints of severe itching** over their entire bodies except for their face; the itching increases **during the night.**
HPI	The male family members also report penile and scrotal skin lesions. The family is of **low socioeconomic status** and lives in a single room under **crowded conditions.**
PE	Papulovesicular lesions; **"burrows"** seen in the dorsal interdigital web spaces and flexor aspects of both wrists; lesions also seen around elbows, anterior axillary folds, periumbilical area, lower buttocks, and thighs; **face was spared; scrotal and penile lesions** seen in male members were **nodular** and reddish.
Labs	**Female adult mite** was seen with a hand lens when teased out of her burrow with a needle.
Imaging	N/A
Gross Pathology	N/A
Micro Pathology	N/A
Treatment	**All family** members need to be treated; **benzyl benzoate,** and **permethrin** are effective; all clothing, linen, etc., must be boiled and washed.
Discussion	Scabies is caused by infestation with *Sarcoptes scabiei,* **a mite** that bores into the corneal layer of the skin, forming burrows in which it deposits its eggs. The scabies organism does not survive for > 48 hours away from the host; thus, **skin-to-skin transfer of organisms** is a more important method of spread than exposure to contaminated bedding or clothing. Outside of institutions, most infestations are transmitted **through sexual contact.**

ID/CC   A 15-day-old **infant** is brought by his mother to the pediatric emergency room in a state of marked **muscle rigidity and spasm.**

HPI   The mother is illiterate and did **not receive any prenatal care**; the delivery was conducted at home and, according to her, was uneventful and full term. The child did **not receive any immunizations**; directed questioning reveals that he has been crying excessively for the past two weeks and has not been feeding normally.

PE   Extremely ill-looking infant in a state of **generalized rigidity and opisthotonus**; on slightest touch or noise, spasm worsens and he develops a stridor and becomes cyanosed.

Labs   Diagnosis is largely clinical; **culture of umbilical stump yields** *Clostridium tetani.*

Imaging   N/A

Gross Pathology   N/A

Micro Pathology   N/A

Treatment   **Ventilatory assistance; supportive** management; maintenance of nutritional, fluid, and electrolyte balance; **tetanus antitoxin;** control of tetanic spasms with diazepam.

Discussion   Tetanus neonatorum accounts for a considerable proportion of infant deaths in developing countries, primarily owing to the **lack of availability of good prenatal care** (no tetanus immunization); untrained birth attendants in rural areas use **contaminated** material to cut or anoint the **umbilical cord.** Tetanus is caused by *Clostridium tetani*, a gram-positive, motile, nonencapsulated. anaerobic, spore-bearing bacillus; its effects are mediated through production of a powerful **neurotoxin (tetanospasmin).** The toxin acts principally on the spinal cord, altering normal control of the reflex arc by suppressing the inhibition regularly mediated by the internuncial neurons.

. . . .

TETANUS NEONATORUM

ID/CC	A 40-year-old male who recently went **hiking in a forest** in the **western U.S.** presents with **symmetric weakness** of the lower extremities that has now progressed over the past few days to involve the trunk and the upper arms.
HPI	The patient does not report any sensory symptoms.
PE	Higher mental functions intact; **symmetric flaccid paralysis** with an **ascending pattern** of spread noted; **no sensory loss** demonstrated; on careful examination of hairy areas of the body, a **tick** was found **embedded in the scalp.**
Labs	LP: CSF normal. EMG: nerve conduction velocity and compound muscle action potentials decreased.
Imaging	N/A
Gross Pathology	N/A
Micro Pathology	N/A
Treatment	Tick was **detached without being squeezed,** and this led to **resolution of symptoms** over the next few days.
Discussion	Feeding ticks may elaborate a **neurotoxin** that causes tick paralysis; symmetric weakness of the lower extremities progresses to an **ascending flaccid paralysis** over several hours to days, although the sensorium remains clear and sensory function is normal. **FIRST AID** p.186

. . . .

TICK PARALYSIS

ID/CC	An 8-year-old male who recently emigrated from India presents with **bilateral eye irritation** and **photophobia**.
HPI	He reports **recurrent episodes** of similar eye irritation and redness **in the past**.
PE	Conjunctival congestion; **multiple (> 5) follicles**, each at least 0.5 mm in diameter, seen **in upper tarsal conjunctiva;** inflammatory thickening of tarsal conjunctiva; new vessels (= PANNUS) seen in cornea at superior limbus; **punctate keratitis**.
Labs	Diagnosis confirmed by demonstration of characteristic cytoplasmic inclusion bodies (= HALBERSTAEDTER–PROWAZEK BODIES) in Giemsa staining of conjunctival scrapings.
Imaging	N/A
Gross Pathology	N/A
Micro Pathology	*Chlamydia trachomatis* is typically seen in conjunctival scrapings in colony form in the epithelial cells as H-P inclusion bodies. Histologically there is lymphocytic infiltration involving the whole adenoid layer of parts of the conjunctiva; special aggregations of lymphocytes form **follicles** that tend to show necrosis and certain large multinucleated cells (= LEBER'S CELLS).
Treatment	Topical **tetracycline** with systemic **tetracycline/doxycycline/erythromycin/azithromycin;** prophylaxis of family contacts with topical tetracycline.
Discussion	*Chlamydia trachomatis* causes a variety of ocular diseases, including **neonatal inclusion conjunctivitis, sporadic inclusion conjunctivitis in adults, and sporadic as well as endemic trachoma;** trachoma is endemic in North Africa, in the Middle East, and among the Native American population of the southwestern United States. In endemic areas, trachoma is transmitted from eye to hand to eye, especially among young children in regions where standards of cleanliness are poor. Sporadic trachoma infection in nonendemic areas as well as sporadic inclusion conjunctivitis in adults results from transmission of the agent from the genital tract to the eye. Trachoma is a **major cause of blindness** in endemic areas. **FIRST AID** p.187

TRACHOMA

ID/CC A 30-year-old soldier who had been admitted for a **gunshot wound** in the right thigh presents with **severe pain and swelling** at the site of his injury.

HPI The patient's right lower limb had become discolored, and several bullae had appeared on the skin. He has passed very little urine over the past day, and the urine he has passed has been dark ("cola-colored").

PE VS: low-grade fever; marked tachycardia. PE: diaphoresis; skin of right thigh discolored (bronze to purple red); site of injury exquisitely tender and tense and **oozing** a thin, dark, and **foul-smelling fluid**; **crepitus** while palpating thigh.

Labs CBC: low hematocrit. Gram stain of exudate and necrotic material at wound site reveals presence of **large gram-positive rods**; anaerobic culture of exudate and blood yields *Clostridium perfringens* type A; culture isolate demonstrates **positive Nagler reaction** (due to presence of alpha toxin lecithinase); further labs confirm presence of **intravascular hemolysis, myo- and hemoglobinuria**, and **acute tubular necrosis**.

Imaging XR-Right Thigh: presence of **gas in soft tissues**.

Gross Pathology Overlying skin purple-bronze, markedly edematous with vesiculobullous changes with little suppurative reaction.

Micro Pathology **Coagulative necrosis**, edema, **gas formation**, and many large **gram-positive bacilli** found in affected muscle tissue; relatively sparse infiltration of PMNs noted in the bordering muscle tissue.

Treatment Surgical debridement; antibiotics (penicillin, clindamycin, tetracycline, metronidazole); hyperbaric oxygen therapy and polyvalent antitoxin; supportive management of associated multiorgan failure.

Discussion A rapidly progressive myonecrosis caused by *Clostridium perfringens* type A, it develops in a wound with low oxygen tension (embedded foreign bodies containing calcium or silicates cause lowering of oxygen tension, leading to germination of the spores). The most important toxin is the alpha toxin lecithinase, which produces hemolysis and myonecrosis.

. . . .

TRAUMATIC GAS GANGRENE

ID/CC   A 10-year-old child who lives in tropical Africa presents with multiple papillomatous skin lesions and pain in both legs.

HPI   The first lesion had appeared on the leg as a small indurated papule that ulcerated into a granulomatous papilloma.

PE   Multiple papillomatous skin lesions seen, especially in intertriginous areas; lesions were painless and exuding a serous fluid; painful hyperkeratotic lesions seen on palms and soles; both tibia were tender to palpation.

Labs   Dark-field microscopic examination of exudate from lesions established the diagnosis by revealing organisms with the characteristic morphology and rotational motion of pathogenic treponemes; nontreponemal serologic tests (i.e., VDRL and RPR tests) and treponemal tests (i.e., FTA-ABS test) were positive.

Imaging   XR-Legs: evidence of periostitis of the tibia.

Gross Pathology   N/A

Micro Pathology   N/A

Treatment   Long-acting intramuscular benzathine penicillin G is the treatment of choice.

Discussion   Yaws, the most common of the nonvenereal treponematoses, is a chronic infection of skin and bones caused by *T. pertenue.* Yaws occurs in tropical areas of Africa, Asia, and Central and South America; it is principally a disease of childhood, and initial infection occurs between 5 and 15 years of age. Transmission is by direct contact with infected skin lesions containing treponemes and is fostered by conditions of overcrowding and poor hygiene. The disease may occur in three stages: primary, secondary, and tertiary. Only lesions of primary and secondary yaws are infectious.

· ·

YAWS

ID/CC	A **15-year-old male** who resides in Florida presents with **nausea** and vomiting, **fever**, and **marked neck stiffness**.
HPI	He also complains of a severe bifrontal headache. Careful history reveals that he **swam for several hours in brackish water** approximately a week ago.
PE	VS: fever; tachycardia. PE: signs of meningeal irritation (neck rigidity, positive Kernig's sign and Brudzinski's sign); funduscopy reveals mild papilledema.
Labs	LP: bloody CSF (raised RBC count may also be due to examiner's inability to recognize proliferating amebas) shows intense neutrophilia, pleocytosis, high protein, and low sugar; no organism seen on Gram, ZN, or India ink staining of CSF; **wet preparation** of CSF reveals viable *Naegleria* **trophozoites**; diagnosis confirmed using direct fluorescent antibody staining.
Imaging	N/A
Gross Pathology	Lesions are mostly present in the olfactory nerves and brain. Focal hemorrhages, extensive fibrinoid necrosis, and blood vessel thrombosis with nerve tissue necrosis.
Micro Pathology	*Naegleria fowleri* trophozoites seen as 10- to 20-um-diameter organisms with large nucleus, small granular cytoplasm, distinct ectoplasm, and bulbous pseudopodia.
Treatment	Intracisternal and IV **amphotericin B**, miconazole, rifampin; prognosis is very poor.
Discussion	Primary amebic meningoencephalitis is caused by amebas of the genus *Naegleria* or *Acanthamoeba.* The former most often affects children and young adults, appears to be acquired by swimming in warm, fresh/brackish water, and is almost always fatal, with the ameba gaining entry into the arachnoid space through the nasal cribriform plate. *Acanthamoeba* infections involve older, immunocompromised individuals and are sometimes characterized by spontaneous recovery.

· ·

AMEBIC MENINGOENCEPHALITIS

ID/CC	A 10-year-old female presents with a **high fever, headache, vomiting,** and impaired consciousness.
HPI	She suffered a generalized **seizure** about 45 minutes ago. She was previously diagnosed with **cyanotic congenital heart disease** (ventricular septal defect with Eisenmenger's syndrome).
PE	VS: fever. PE: altered sensorium; **papilledema;** nuchal rigidity; clubbing; **central cyanosis;** cardiac auscultation suggestive of VSD with severe pulmonary arterial hypertension.
Labs	Blood culture reveals **mixed infection** with *Bacteroides,* microaerophilic streptococci, *S. aureus,* and *Klebsiella;* staining and culture of pus aspirated from brain abscess confirm polymicrobial infection.
Imaging	CT (with contrast): multiple ring-enhancing lesions with low attenuation centers (= ABSCESS) surrounding cerebral edema and ventricular compression.
Gross Pathology	Cavity filled with thick, liquefied pus surrounded by fibrous capsule of variable thickness; pericapsular zone of gliosis and edema.
Micro Pathology	Central portion contains degenerated PMNs and cellular debris; capsule is composed of collagenous fibrous tissue with blood vessels and mixed inflammatory cells.
Treatment	High-dose, extended parenteral broad-spectrum antibiotic coverage; **CT-directed drainage of pus.**
Discussion	Brain abscesses arise secondary to **hematogenous spread** from another infection (bronchiectasis, endocarditis), from contiguous spread from adjacent infection (chronic otitis media, mastoiditis, sinusitis), or following **direct implantation** from trauma. Patients with congenital heart disease with right-to-left shunt are particularly predisposed because the normal filtering action of the pulmonary vasculature is lost.

. . . .

BRAIN ABSCESS WITH CYANOTIC HEART DISEASE

ID/CC	A 30-year-old male presents with a **high fever** and chills, **headache, nausea,** vomiting, and muscle aches.
HPI	Yesterday he had an episode involving abnormal movements of his right hand and face (= FOCAL SEIZURE). He also has difficulty comprehending speech and has **olfactory hallucinations.** He has no history of psychiatric illness.
PE	VS: fever; tachycardia; mild tachypnea; normotension. PE: **confused and disoriented; papilledema;** mild nuchal rigidity; Kernig's sign positive; paraphasic errors in speech; deep tendon reflexes normal and bilaterally symmetric.
Labs	LP: cells 400/uL with **mononuclear pleocytosis;** mildly elevated protein; normal glucose; CSF PCR reveals **herpes simplex virus type 1 (HSV-1);** serum complement-fixing antibody titer > 1:1000. EEG: **spiked and slow waves localized to temporal lobes.**
Imaging	CT: characteristic changes of **encephalitis** seen over **temporal lobes.**
Gross Pathology	Hemorrhagic, necrotizing encephalitis most severe along inferior and medial regions of temporal lobes and orbitofrontal gyri.
Micro Pathology	Brain biopsy reveals **Cowdry intranuclear viral inclusion bodies** in both neurons and glial cells with perivascular inflammatory infiltrates.
Treatment	**Intravenous acyclovir.**
Discussion	Herpes simplex virus is the **most common cause of acute sporadic encephalitis** in the United States. In the newborn, HSV-2 is usually the cause; after the neonatal period, most cases result from HSV-1. Neonatal infection (usually HSV-2) occurs after exposure to maternal genital infection at the time of delivery. The precise pathogenesis of HSV-1 encephalitis in the older child or the adult is not clear, but viral spread into the temporal lobe by both olfactory and trigeminal routes has been postulated. **FIRST AID** p.201

. . . .

HERPES SIMPLEX ENCEPHALITIS

ID/CC	An 11-year-old girl is brought to the ER with high **fever, chills, severe headache, vomiting,** and obtundation.
HPI	Her parents report that she suffered a generalized **seizure** about an hour ago. A few days ago, the family had returned from a summer vacation in **south India,** where the child often **played in irrigated rice farms.** She **did not receive any immunizations** prior to her travel.
PE	VS: fever. PE: patient is stuporous; neck stiffness and Kernig's sign positive (due to meningeal irritation); mild papilledema; tremors noted in hands.
Labs	LP: CSF reveals pleocytosis with **predominant lymphocytosis, mildly elevated proteins, and normal sugar** (suggestive of aseptic meningitis); IgM enzyme immunoassay performed on acute and convalescent sera and CSF reveals significant titer of antibodies to **Japanese encephalitis** virus.
Imaging	CT-Head: areas of **low density in the thalamus and basal ganglia.**
Gross Pathology	N/A
Micro Pathology	N/A
Treatment	Supportive; experimental intrathecal alpha-interferon therapy.
Discussion	Japanese encephalitis virus is a **flavivirus** that causes **disease in humans, horses and pigs.** It is **widely distributed in Asia** from Japan and Eastern Siberia to Indonesia and westward to India; **epidemics** occur in **summer months** coincident with the abundance of the **mosquito vector** *Culex tritaeniorhychnus.* The vector breeds in irrigated rice fields and bites preferentially at sunset and sunrise; **pigs are the amplifying hosts,** whereas man is the incidental "dead-end" host. A **vaccine is available** for routine use for childhood immunization in Japan and in developed countries to protect travelers.

. . . .

JAPANESE ENCEPHALITIS

ID/CC	A **neonate died** shortly after birth.
HPI	Review of the medical record reveals history of **refusal to feed,** an extensive **maculopapular skin rash** on his legs and trunk, **respiratory distress,** diarrhea, and seizures shortly after birth.
PE	N/A
Labs	N/A
Imaging	N/A
Gross Pathology	N/A
Micro Pathology	N/A
Treatment	N/A
Discussion	Neonatal listeriosis may occur early or late in neonatal life. Infants may be acutely ill at birth and may die within hours as a result of disseminated listeriosis, which is also called **granulomatosis infantiseptica.** This condition is characterized by **hepatosplenomegaly, thrombocytopenia,** generalized **skin papules,** whitish pharyngeal patches, and **pneumonia.** Commonly, a stained smear of meconium will reveal **gram-positive bacilli,** suggesting the diagnosis.

. . . .

LISTERIA MENINGITIS

ID/CC   A 30-year-old male **laboratory researcher** presents with a **high fever, neck rigidity,** retro-orbital pain, and severe myalgias of a few days' duration.

HPI   The patient also complains of a **sore throat** and photophobia. His work in the lab involves **close contact with** experimental animals such as **hamsters, white mice, and nude mice.** He was adequately vaccinated.

PE   VS: fever. PE: neck stiffness and **Kernig's sign positive** (due to meningeal irritation); pharyngeal inflammation but no exudate noted.

Labs   CBC: mild leukopenia. LP: CSF suggestive of **aseptic meningitis; LCM virus isolated** from CSF. IgG and IgM antibodies detected in serum by immunofluorescent assay.

Imaging   N/A

Gross Pathology   N/A

Micro Pathology   N/A

Treatment   Supportive; ribavirin may play a role.

Discussion   Lymphochoriomeningitis virus is an **arenavirus.** Sporadic cases occur after **infection with feral mice,** but the **most common sources** of human infection are **pet/lab rodents.** The virus is considered a **major lab hazard,** and care must be taken to avoid accidental infection. There is **no** commercially available **vaccine.**

. . . .

LYMPHOCYTIC CHORIOMENINGITIS

ID/CC	A 26-year-old nurse presented with headaches and **recent-onset seizures**; she also complained of increasing **right-sided numbness and blurring of vision.**
HPI	A clinical diagnosis of HSV encephalitis had previously been made, for which the patient was treated with two courses of acyclovir without any amelioration of symptoms; the **disease continued to progress** both radiologically and clinically. On serology she tested **HIV positive.**
PE	Neurologic exam reveals **cognitive mental impairment; visual field defects and sensory dysphasia** seen; **an ill-defined sensory loss** on right side of body.
Labs	HIV positive by ELISA and Western blot.
Imaging	MR (T2-weighted): patchy high-intensity lesions **in the deep white matter of left cerebral hemisphere** involving temporal, parietal, and occipital lobes.
Gross Pathology	N/A
Micro Pathology	Stereotactic biopsy sections show abnormal brain with rarefaction, numerous reactive astrocytes, foamy histiocytes, and inflammatory infiltrate around some vessels; **JC virus in situ hybridization** shows many **positive nuclei;** no herpesvirus inclusions seen; **electron microscopy** demonstrates cells with **typical papovavirus** structures in nucleus.
Treatment	Disease was **relentlessly progressive** and resulted in **death within six months.**
Discussion	Progressive multifocal leukoencephalopathy is a **progressive demyelinating disease related to JC papovavirus infection;** the largest number of cases occur in **persons who are immunocompromised** for any of a variety of reasons, including organ transplantation, hematologic and other malignant diseases, chronic immunosuppressive therapy, and AIDS.

. . . .

PROGRESSIVE MULTIFOCAL LEUKOENCEPHALOPATHY

ID/CC	A 30-year-old male is seen with complaints of a **rash** along with **pain in his left ear** and inability to move the muscles of his face with accompanying asymmetry.
HPI	He suffered an attack of **chickenpox during childhood** but has no history either of a similar rash over his face or of any visual symptoms (to rule out herpes zoster ophthalmicus).
PE	**Vesicular rash** over left pinna (= OTITIS EXTERNA); left-sided lower motor neuron–type **facial nerve palsy** (patient is unable to frown and unable to blink left eye; eyeballs roll up during attempt to close eye; patient is unable to whistle; taste sensation over anterior two-thirds of tongue lost on left side).
Labs	Although the diagnosis is predominantly clinical, a **Tzanck test** examining lesion scrapings (showing evidence of multinucleate acantholytic cells), direct culture, and immunohistochemical identification of infected cells allow identification of the virus.
Imaging	N/A
Gross Pathology	Neuritis and vesicular skin lesions confined to distribution of geniculate ganglion of facial nerve.
Micro Pathology	Vesicular skin lesions with **herpes viral inclusions,** i.e., intranuclear, acidophil inclusions with a halo around them (= COWDRY TYPE A INCLUSIONS); syncytial cells also seen.
Treatment	**Systemic steroids** are mainstay of management.
Discussion	**Herpes zoster** of the **geniculate ganglion,** or Ramsay Hunt syndrome, presents as a vesicular rash on the pinna followed by ipsilateral LMN facial nerve palsy.

RAMSAY HUNT SYNDROME

ID/CC	A **6-year-old** boy is brought by his parents to the emergency room in a comatose state.
HPI	The child was suffering from **chickenpox** and had been given **aspirin** for fever by the family physician.
PE	VS: fever. PE: **comatose** with papulovesicular rash all over body; fundus shows marked papilledema; no icterus; **hepatomegaly.**
Labs	**Impaired liver function; blood ammonia** concentration increased; AST and ALT levels elevated; PT prolonged; **serum bilirubin normal.** LP (done after controlling raised ICT): normal spinal fluid.
Imaging	CT: generalized **cerebral edema**, decreased density of white matter.
Gross Pathology	N/A
Micro Pathology	Liver biopsy reveals **microvesicular steatosis** with little or no inflammation; electron microscopy shows marked **mitochondrial abnormalities.**
Treatment	Specific therapy is not available. Supportive measures for **management of hepatic encephalopathy** include lactulose to control hyperammonemia, fresh frozen plasma to replenish clotting factors, mannitol or dexamethasone to lower increased intracranial pressure, and mechanical ventilation.
Discussion	Although the cause of Reye's syndrome is unknown, epidemiologic evidence strongly links this disorder with outbreaks of **viral disease, especially influenza and chickenpox.** Epidemiologic evidence has also prompted the Surgeon General and the American Academy of Pediatrics Committee on Infectious Diseases to recommend that **salicylates not be given to children with chickenpox or influenza.**

REYE'S SYNDROME

ID/CC	A 30-year-old male presents with a **high fever, neck stiffness,** and **drowsiness.**
HPI	He also complains of nausea and vomiting. He **recently traveled** along the **Mississippi–Ohio River basin.**
PE	VS: fever. PE: **neck stiffness** and **Kernig's sign positive** (due to meningeal irritation); right oculomotor nerve palsy noted; mild papilledema.
Labs	IgM enzyme immunoassay done on paired sera, and CSF confirms the diagnosis of **St. Louis virus** infection. LP: CSF exam reveals pleocytosis with predominant lymphocytosis suggestive of **aseptic meningitis.**
Imaging	N/A
Gross Pathology	N/A
Micro Pathology	Inflammation and neuronal degeneration, principally in the thalamus, midbrain, and brainstem.
Treatment	Supportive treatment.
Discussion	St. Louis encephalitis virus is the **most common cause of epidemic encephalitis** in the United States; cases occur annually as isolated events or in summer–autumn encephalitis epidemics. **Most** infections **are asymptomatic.** The disease occurs throughout the U.S., but outbreaks have also occurred in the Caribbean as well as in Central and South America. **FIRST AID** p.198

ST. LOUIS ENCEPHALITIS

ID/CC The case of a **12-year-old boy** who **died of a progressive degenerative neurologic disease** was discussed at an autopsy meeting.

HPI The child had been developing normally up to 10 years of age, when his teachers noted a **progressive deterioration in intellect and personality**; this was followed by the development of **seizures akin to myoclonus**, signs of pyramidal and extrapyramidal disease, and finally a **state of decerebrate rigidity**. The child **died seven months after the onset** of symptoms. His history revealed that he had had a **severe attack of measles at the age of two**.

PE N/A

Labs LP: routine CSF profile normal. **Gamma globulin level elevated**; markedly **elevated levels of measles antibody** present in both serum and CSF; despite the elevated antibody titers, **antibody to the M protein was not present**. EEG: pattern of **burst suppression and biphasic sharp and slow waves**.

Imaging MR: nonspecific parenchymal abnormalities.

Gross Pathology N/A

Micro Pathology Histopathologically, the encephalitis involved both white and gray matter and was marked by lymphocytic infiltration, nerve cell degeneration, and demyelination; measles antigen demonstrated by immunofluorescence analysis, and particles resembling paramyxovirus were detected by electron microscopy.

Treatment No specific therapy available.

Discussion Subacute sclerosing panencephalitis is caused by a **defective** (major defect is the lack or altered expression of the M-matrix protein) form of **measles virus** (family Paramyxoviridae); SSPE is a **late complication of a measles** infection that is not eliminated from the host. Immunization against measles is the only effective preventive tool.
FIRST AID p.198

· ·

SUBACUTE SCLEROSING PANENCEPHALITIS (SSPE)

ID/CC A **6-year-old male** being treated for **primary pulmonary tuberculosis** presents with **diplopia,** increasing drowsiness, irritability, and unexplained, recurrent **vomiting.**

HPI The child has had a low-grade fever, loss of appetite, and a persistent headache over the past few weeks.

PE VS: fever. PE: stuporous; signs of meningeal irritation noted (**neck rigidity, Kernig's sign**); **CN III and IV palsy** on right side; funduscopy reveals **papilledema.**

Labs LP (guarded): CSF under **increased pressure** and **turbid;** on standing, a "**cobweb" coagulum** formed at center of tube; CSF studies reveal **lymphocytic pleocytosis,** greatly **elevated protein,** and **low sugar;** ZN staining of CSF coagulum reveals presence of **acid-fast bacilli;** radiometric culture yields *Mycobacterium tuberculosis.*

Imaging CT: suggests **basal exudates, inflammatory granulomas,** and a **communicating hydrocephalus;** striking meningeal enhancement noted in post-contrast studies.

Gross Pathology Meningeal surface covered with yellowish-gray exudates and tubercles that are most numerous at base of brain and along the course of the middle cerebral artery; subarachnoid space and arachnoid villi obliterated (leading to poor absorption of CSF and hence a communicating hydrocephalus).

Micro Pathology Subarachnoid space contains gelatinous exudate of chronic inflammatory cells, obliterating cisterns, and encasing cranial nerves; well-formed **granulomas** occasionally seen, most often at base of brain; arteries running through subarachnoid space show "obliterative endarteritis."

Treatment Antituberculous therapy with rifampin, isoniazid, ethambutol and pyrazinamide; steroids; ventriculoperitoneal shunt to relieve hydrocephalus.

Discussion Tuberculous infection reaches the meninges through the hematogenous route, resulting in a clinically subacute form of meningitis; it is often complicated by cranial nerve palsies, a communicating hydrocephalus, decerebrate posturing, convulsions, coma, and death.

TUBERCULAR MENINGITIS

ID/CC	A 25-year-old **recently married woman** is concerned about a scanty, offensively **malodorous vaginal discharge**.
HPI	She states that the discharge is **thin, grayish-white, and foul-smelling**. She does not complain of vulvar pruritus or soreness.
PE	Pelvic exam confirms presence of a homogenous, grayish-white, watery discharge adherent to the vaginal walls that yields a "fishy" odor when mixed with KOH; no injection and excoriation of the vulva, vagina, or cervix.
Labs	Vaginal pH > 5; saline smear reveals presence of **characteristic "clue cells"** (squamous epithelial cells with smudged borders due to adherent bacteria).
Imaging	N/A
Gross Pathology	N/A
Micro Pathology	N/A
Treatment	Single dose of **metronidazole** (2 g) effective in treating the infection. Oral clindamycin is an alternative drug.
Discussion	Although bacterial vaginitis was originally thought to be caused by *Gardnerella vaginalis,* this organism is now recognized to be part of the normal vaginal flora. Bacterial vaginosis is now known to result from a **synergistic interaction of bacteria** in which the normal *Lactobacillus* species in the vagina is ultimately replaced by **high concentrations of anaerobic bacteria,** including *Bacteroides, Peptostreptococcus, Peptococcus,* and *Mobiluncus* species along with a markedly greater number of *G. vaginalis* organisms than is encountered in normal vaginal secretions. Bacterial vaginosis is known to increase the risk of pelvic inflammatory disease, chorioamnionitis, and premature birth.

. . . .

BACTERIAL VAGINOSIS

ID/CC	A 25-year-old puerpera who was **lactating** her week-old infant presents with **pain and swelling** in her left breast.
HPI	The symptoms commenced acutely, and she does not recall any previous breast lumps or swellings.
PE	**Skin overlying** left breast is **red, edematous, tender, and hot**; area of tense induration felt underlying inflamed skin.
Labs	Culture of pus drained from **breast abscess** and **nasopharyngeal swab** taken from the infant **grew** *S. aureus*.
Imaging	USG: nearly anechoic area with posterior enhancement.
Gross Pathology	N/A
Micro Pathology	N/A
Treatment	**Penicillinase-resistant antibiotic; incision** (in a radial direction over the affected segment) **and dependent drainage** of intramammary abscess; breast feeding was temporarily discontinued.
Discussion	Bacterial mastitis most commonly occurs in lactating women due to infection of a hematoma or secondary infection of plasma cell mastitis; the infecting **organism is mostly penicillin-resistant** *Staphylococcus aureus*.

BREAST ABSCESS

ID/CC	A 28-year-old primigravida at 36 weeks' gestation presents with a **high fever**.
HPI	She was being monitored following a **premature rupture of the membranes**.
PE	VS: **fever**; fetal tachycardia. PE: **uterine tenderness**.
Labs	Elevated maternal total lymphocyte count; **vaginal swab culture revealed colonization with group B streptococcus**.
Imaging	N/A
Gross Pathology	N/A
Micro Pathology	N/A
Treatment	Presence of group B streptococcus in vagina after premature rupture of membranes was an indication for **immediate delivery and treatment of the infant**; mother was also treated with **intravenous antibiotics**.
Discussion	A significant proportion of the population is colonized in the vagina and rectum with **group B streptococcus, which is correlated with preterm labor, premature rupture of membranes** (PROM), **chorioamnionitis, and neonatal sepsis**; neonates with group B streptococcus sepsis have a 25% mortality rate. Among preterm neonates, this figure doubles to over 50%; therefore **antibiotic prophylaxis** is recommended in the setting of **preterm delivery and PROM** even without the diagnosis of frank chorioamnionitis. When chorioamnionitis is suspected, intravenous antibiotics are started and delivery is hastened.

· ·

CHORIOAMNIONITIS

ID/CC	An 8-month-old male infant is brought to a pediatrician because of severe, intractable **chronic diarrhea** and **failure to thrive.**
HPI	The **mother died of AIDS** shortly after the baby was delivered. The baby was **asymptomatic at birth.**
PE	VS: fever; tachycardia. PE: emaciated, grossly malnourished; **oral thrush; generalized lymphadenopathy; hepatosplenomegaly.**
Labs	**Decreased CD4+ cell count;** increased serum immunoglobulin level with impaired production of specific antibodies; **ELISA and Western blot for HIV-1 positive** (could be due to placental transfer of antibodies to HIV, but strongly supports diagnosis in presence of symptoms); PCR for **HIV RNA positive** (confirming HIV infection).
Imaging	N/A
Gross Pathology	N/A
Micro Pathology	N/A
Treatment	Nutritional support, *Pneumocystis carinii* prophylaxis, azidothymidine (= ZIDOVUDINE, or AZT) therapy (suppresses replication by inhibiting viral reverse transcriptase), and anti-infective agents for specific infections; IV serum immunoglobulin to reduce frequency of bacterial infections; **oral polio vaccine and BCG contraindicated.**
Discussion	Vertical transmission of HIV-1 may occur in utero through **transplacental passage** of the virus, **during delivery,** or **postnatally through breast feeding;** however, it is believed that most infections are acquired at birth through contact with contaminated blood or secretions. Women who carry the virus should thus be discouraged from becoming pregnant or from breast feeding. The rate of transmission of HIV-1 from mother to infant has varied from 13% to 45%, with an average of 25%; however, when AZT is administered to HIV-1-infected pregnant women and to infants during the first six weeks of life, the risk of maternal–infant transmission is significantly reduced.

· ·

HIV TRANSMISSION IN PREGNANCY

ID/CC	A 28-year-old **sexually active woman** presents with crampy **lower abdominal pain,** yellowish **vaginal discharge,** and general malaise.
HPI	She also complains of continuous low-grade fever and reveals that the **pain is exacerbated during and immediately after menstruation** (= CONGESTIVE DYSMENORRHEA). She uses a copper **intrauterine device** for contraception.
PE	VS: low-grade fever. PE: **lower abdominal tenderness;** bimanual pelvic exam demonstrates **purulent vaginal discharge,** bilateral **adnexal tenderness,** and pain on movement of cervix (= MUCOPURULENT CERVICITIS).
Labs	CBC: leukocytosis with left shift. Increased ESR; endocervical swab sent for microscopic exam, staining and culture revealed combined infection with *Neisseria gonorrhoeae* (cultured on Thayer–Martin medium) and *Chlamydia trachomatis* (identified on cell culture, immunofluorescence, and antigen capture assay); **laparoscopy** ("gold standard" for diagnosis) confirmed diagnosis.
Imaging	USG: free pelvic fluid, dilated tubular structure in adnexa.
Gross Pathology	Erythema and swelling of fallopian tubes on laparoscopy; seropurulent exudate noted on surface of tubes from fimbriated end.
Micro Pathology	Endocervical swab reveals increased neutrophils and gram-negative diplococci seen both intra- and extracellularly; cervical biopsy reveals inclusions containing *Chlamydia* within columnar cells.
Treatment	Antibiotic therapy with cefoxitin (for *N. gonorrhoeae*) and doxycycline (for chlamydial infection); male partners must be treated for STDs.
Discussion	Pelvic inflammatory disease usually occurs as a primary infection that ascends from the lower genital tract due to STDs caused by *Neisseria gonorrhoeae* and *Chlamydia trachomatis.* Sequelae of PID include peritonitis; intestinal obstruction due to adhesions; dissemination leading to arthritis, meningitis, and endocarditis; chronic pelvic pain; infertility; ectopic pregnancy; and recurrent PID. **FIRST AID** p.192

· ·

PELVIC INFLAMMATORY DISEASE (PID)

ID/CC	A 30-year-old **woman** presents to the ER with an abrupt-onset **high fever, vomiting, profuse diarrhea,** severe muscle aches, and disorientation.
HPI	One day ago she developed an **extensive skin rash** all over her body. Her husband says she used a **vaginal sponge** for contraception.
PE	VS: fever; tachycardia; hypotension. PE: extremely toxic-looking; drowsy but responding to verbal commands; **extensive scarlatiniform rash** seen involving entire body; pharyngeal, conjunctival, and vaginal mucosa congested (frank hyperemia); no neck rigidity or Kernig's sign demonstrable; funduscopic exam normal; no localizing neurologic deficits.
Labs	CBC: leukocytosis; thrombocytopenia. UA: mild pyuria (in absence of UTI). BUN and creatinine elevated; blood cultures sterile; **culture of cervical secretions grows *S. aureus*.** LP: CSF normal. Serology for Rocky mountain spotted fever, leptospirosis, and measles negative.
Imaging	N/A
Gross Pathology	N/A
Micro Pathology	N/A
Treatment	**Vigorous IV fluids** and parenteral **penicillinase-resistant penicillin** or first-generation cephalosporins; patient in this case recovered, and typical skin desquamation was seen over palms and soles during convalescence.
Discussion	Toxic shock syndrome results from infection with *S. aureus*. Its effects are mediated through the **exotoxin TSST-1,** which functions as a superantigen, stimulating the production of interleukin-1 and tumor necrosis factor. Staphylococcal TSS has been associated with the use of **vaginal contraceptive sponges** and with many types of localized staphylococcal soft tissue infections. Most cases of TSS occur in **menstruating women.**

TOXIC SHOCK SYNDROME (TSS)

ID/CC   A **20-year-old Asian woman** presents with complaints of **infertility** and **heavy bleeding during menses** (= MENORRHAGIA).

HPI   She was treated for **pulmonary tuberculosis** a few years ago. She has been unable to conceive despite unprotected intercourse for the past two years. Her husband's semen analysis is normal.

PE   On pelvic exam, small, fixed **adnexal masses** are palpable that are matted and fixed to uterus (= "FROZEN PELVIS").

Labs   Culture of endometrial curettings yields *Mycobacterium tuberculosis;* histologic examination of curettings reveals presence of **characteristic tubercles**; Mantoux skin test strongly positive.

Imaging   CXR: left apical fibrosis (evidence of old healed pulmonary tuberculosis). (Hysterosalpingography [HSG] is contraindicated in a proven case of tuberculosis. When done in asymptomatic cases, HSG yields certain typical findings, including a **rigid, nonperistaltic, pipelike tube**; beading and variation in filling density; **calcification** of the tube; **cornual block; jagged fluffiness of the tubal outline**; and vascular or lymphatic extravasation of the dye.)

Gross Pathology   Tubes are enlarged, thickened, and tortuous; examination of uterus reveals evidence of **synechiae and adhesions** (leading to **Asherman's syndrome**).

Micro Pathology   Microscopic exam of tubes, ovaries, and endometrium reveals evidence of **granulomas** with giant cells and **caseation**.

Treatment   Four-drug therapy with isoniazid, pyrazinamide, ethambutol, and rifampicin; pyridoxine to prevent isoniazid-induced deficiency.

Discussion   Genital tuberculosis is almost always secondary to a focus elsewhere in the body, with the bloodstream by far the most common method of spread. The fallopian tubes are the most frequently involved part of the genital tract, followed by the uterus. Ninety percent of patients are cured with chemotherapy, although only 10% regain fertility.

· ·

TUBERCULAR SALPINGITIS

ID/CC	A 25-year-old male presents with complaints of sudden-onset **fever** and chills, urgency and burning on micturition (= DYSURIA), and perineal pain.
HPI	His symptoms developed a day after he underwent **urethral dilatation** for a stricture.
PE	VS: fever. PE: suprapubic tenderness; rectal exam reveals asymmetrically **swollen**, firm, markedly **tender, hot prostate**; prostatic massage is avoided owing to risk of inducing bacteremia; epididymitis and extreme pain.
Labs	Examination and culture of urine and prostatic secretions reveal infection with *E. coli.*
Imaging	N/A
Gross Pathology	Edematous gland enlargement with suppuration of entire gland, possibly abscesses and focal areas of necrosis that have coalesced.
Micro Pathology	Initially minimal leukocytic infiltration of stroma. Later, necrosis of the gland may lead to gland fibrosis.
Treatment	Antibiotic therapy as directed by urine and blood culture sensitivity tests.
Discussion	*E. coli* **is the most common cause;** many cases **follow** the use of **instrumentation for the urethra** and prostate (e.g., catheterization, cystoscopy, urethral dilatation, transurethral resection). Remaining infections are caused by *Klebsiella, Proteus, Pseudomonas,* and *Serratia.* Among the gram positives, enterococcus and *S. aureus* are frequent causative organisms.

· ·

ACUTE PROSTATITIS

ID/CC	A 65-year-old male complains of recurrent burning, urgency, and frequency of micturition together with vague lower abdominal, lumbar, and perineal pain.
HPI	He also complains of a mucoid urethral discharge. He was previously diagnosed via ultrasound with benign prostatic hypertrophy but does not report any severe symptoms of prostatism; his medical history reveals frequent UTIs due to *E. coli.*
PE	VS: stable; no fever. PE: rectal exam reveals enlarged, nodular prostate; biopsy obtained to rule out carcinoma.
Labs	Examination and culture of expressed prostatic secretions reveal leukocytosis and *E. coli.*
Imaging	IVP/Voiding Cystourethrogram (to rule out underlying anatomic cause): normal.
Gross Pathology	Enlarged prostate with nodularity and calculi.
Micro Pathology	Chronic inflammation and few PMNs around glands and ducts on biopsy; dilated ducts containing inspissated secretions (= CORPORA AMYLACEA).
Treatment	Antibiotics (SMX–TMP, carbenicillin, quinolones). High fluid intake and abstinence from alcohol. Recurrences are common.
Discussion	Bacterial prostatitis is usually caused by the same gram-negative bacilli that cause UTIs in females; 80% or more of such infections are caused by *E. coli.* Chronic bacterial prostatitis is common in elderly males with prostatic hyperplasia and is a frequent cause of recurrent UTIs in males (most antibiotics poorly penetrate the prostate; hence the bacteria are not totally eradicated and continuously seed the urinary tract).

· ·

CHRONIC PROSTATITIS

ID/CC	A **28-year-old man** comes to the ER with gradually worsening and now severe **scrotal swelling** and pain radiating to the inguinal area.
HPI	The patient has no significant medical history. He reports pain on urination (due to concomitant urethritis) and notes that he is sexually active with multiple partners. He also notes that the pain is greater on standing and walking and is relieved by rest and elevation of the legs.
PE	VS: normal. PE: **scrotal edema** and erythema; **right epididymis enlarged and tender;** induration present; **elevation** of scrotal contents **relieves pain** (= PREHN'S SIGN).
Labs	UA: pyuria. Culture negative; biopsy of epididymis inoculated into cell cultures grows *Chlamydia trachomatis;* immunofluorescence reveals **subtype D.**
Imaging	US: hypoechoic, enlarged epididymis with hypervascularity.
Gross Pathology	Nonspecific inflammation characterized by congestion and edema.
Micro Pathology	Early stage of the infection is limited to the interstitial connective tissue with white cell infiltration.
Treatment	Antibiotics like doxycycline, minocycline for chlamydia. Course of ofloxacin covers all possibilities of causative organisms.
Discussion	Differentiate from testicular torsion and tumor (scrotal ultrasonography or isotopic flow study may be needed for differentiating). Transmitted sexually in young adults and most often **caused by** *C. trachomatis* **subtypes D–K** and *Neisseria gonorrhoeae.* In those older than 40, *E. coli* and *Pseudomonas* cause most infections. If associated with rectal intercourse, it may be due to Enterobacteriaceae.

· ·

EPIDIDYMITIS

ID/CC	A **10-year-old child** presents with complaints of acute-onset voiding of **tea-colored urine** and **reduced urinary output.**
HPI	The child was treated one week ago for **streptococcal pyoderma** that was confirmed by culture. He also complains of puffiness around the eyes and mild swelling of both feet.
PE	VS: **hypertension** (BP 140/96); fever; tachycardia. PE: periorbital swelling; mild pitting **pedal edema;** no ascites or kidney mass palpable.
Labs	CBC: mild leukocytosis. Elevated BUN and creatinine; **elevated ASO titer;** serum cryoglobulins present. UA: **RBC casts; proteinuria. C3 levels reduced** in blood.
Imaging	N/A
Gross Pathology	Smooth, reddish-brown cortical surface with numerous petechial hemorrhages.
Micro Pathology	Biopsy shows **diffuse glomerulonephritis** resulting from proliferation of endothelial, mesangial, and epithelial cells; granular, **"starry-sky" pattern** of IgG, IgM, and C3 on immunofluorescence; electron microscopy shows **subepithelial "humplike" deposits** (antigen-antibody complexes).
Treatment	Penicillin if still infected with *Streptococcus;* diuretics, salt and water restriction and antihypertensives.
Discussion	Poststreptococcal glomerulonephritis is a classic immune complex–mediated entity that is associated with acute nephritic syndrome, which develops following infection with nephritogenic group A beta-hemolytic streptococci (e.g., types 1, 4, and 12, which are associated with pharyngitis, and types 49, 55, and 57, which are associated with impetigo).

ID/CC A 12-year-old **immigrant from the Middle East** presents with **terminal hematuria,** dysuria, and increased frequency of micturition.

HPI He remembers having played and **bathed in snail-infested streams** while he was in his native country; on one occasion he had developed an **intensely pruritic skin eruption** after bathing in one such stream (= "CERCARIAL DERMATITIS").

PE Pallor noted.

Labs UA: **hematuria;** mild proteinuria and sterile **(abacterial) pyuria.** Microscopic exam of urine and rectal biopsy reveals presence of **ellipsoid eggs with a sharp terminal spine** containing a miracidium surrounded by a thick, rigid shell.

Imaging XR: bladder wall calcification.

Gross Pathology N/A

Micro Pathology N/A

Treatment **Praziquantel,** metrifonate.

Discussion **Three major species** exist. *Schistosoma mansoni, S. japonicum,* and *S. haematobium* infect humans. *S. mansoni* is found in Africa, the Arabian Peninsula, South America, and parts of the Caribbean; *S. japonicum* is found in Japan, China, and the Philippines; and *S. haematobium* **is found in Africa and the Middle East.** Transmission of schistosomiasis **cannot occur in the United States** because of the absence of the specific freshwater **snail that is a intermediary host.** In *S. haematobium* infection, the principal symptoms are terminal hematuria, dysuria, and frequent urination; **hydronephrosis,** pyelonephritis, and **squamous cell carcinoma of the urinary bladder** may develop as **complications.** In *S. mansoni* and *S. japonicum* infection, manifestations may include **fever, malaise, abdominal pain, diarrhea,** or hepatosplenomegaly. Presinusoidal hepatic trapping of eggs and the consequent granulomatous reaction induce **portal hypertension.**

· ·

URINARY SCHISTOSOMIASIS

ID/CC	A 25-year-old **sexually active woman** presents with **burning during micturition** (= DYSURIA), increased frequency and urgency of micturition, and low-grade fever.
HPI	She is otherwise in perfect health.
PE	VS: fever.
Labs	UA: abundant WBCs; mild proteinuria but no casts; staining of sediment reveals presence of gram-positive cocci. Urine culture isolates **coagulase-negative *S. saprophyticus.***
Imaging	N/A
Gross Pathology	N/A
Micro Pathology	N/A
Treatment	Antibiotics (ampicillin, cotrimoxazole, or ciprofloxacin).
Discussion	Enterobacteriaceae like *E. coli, Klebsiella* species, and *Proteus* and *Pseudomonas* species are the most common organisms causing UTI. After *E. coli, S. saprophyticus* is the most common cause of primary nonobstructive UTI in sexually active young women.

· ·

UTI WITH STAPHYLOCOCCUS SAPROPHYTICUS

From the authors of *Underground Clinical Vignettes*

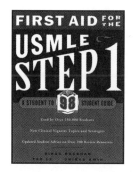

A true classic used by over 200,000 students around the world. The '99 edition features details on the new computerized test, new color plates and thoroughly updated high-yield facts and book reviews. Bi-directional links with the *Underground Clinical Vignettes Step 1* series. ISBN 0-8385-2612-8.

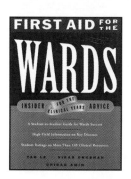

This high-yield student-to-student guide is designed to help students make the transition from the basic sciences to the hospital wards and succeed on their clinical rotations. The book features an orientation to the hospital environment, tips on being an effective and efficient junior medical student, student-proven advice tailored to each core rotation, a database of high-yield clinical facts, and recommendations for clinical pocket books, texts, and references. ISBN 0-8385-2595-4.

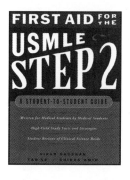

This entirely rewritten second edition now follows in the footsteps of *First Aid for the USMLE Step 1*. Features an exam preparation guide geared to the new computerized test, basic science and clinical high-yield facts, color plates and ratings of USMLE Step 2 books and software. Bi-directional links with the *Underground Clinical Vignettes Step 2* series.

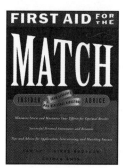

This top rated (5 stars, *Doody Review*) student-to-student guide helps medical students effectively and efficiently navigate the residency application process, helping them make the most of their limited time, money, and energy. The book draws on the advice and experiences of successful student applicants as well as residency directors. Also featured are application and interview tips tailored to each specialty, successful personal statements and CVs with analyses, current trends, and common interview questions with suggested strategies for responding. ISBN 0-8385-2596-2.

The *First Aid* series by Appleton & Lange...the review book leader.
Available through your local health sciences bookstore !

About the Authors

. . . .

VIKAS BHUSHAN, MD

Vikas is a diagnostic radiologist in Los Angeles and the series editor for *Underground Clinical Vignettes*. His interests include traveling, reading, writing, and world music. He is single and can be reached at vbhushan@aol.com

CHIRAG AMIN, MD

Chirag is an orthopedics resident at Orlando Regional Medical Center. He plans on pursuing a spine fellowship. He can be reached at chiragamin@aol.com

TAO LE, MD

Tao is completing a medicine residency at Yale-New Haven Hospital and is applying for a fellowship in allergy and immunology. He is married to Thao, who is a pediatrics resident. He can be reached at taotle@aol.com

VISHAL PALL, MBBS

Vishal recently completed medical school and internship in Chandigarh, India. He hopes to begin his Internal Medicine residency training in the US in July 1999. He can be reached at vishalpall@hotmail.com

HOANG NGUYEN

Hoang (Henry) is a third-year medical student at Northwestern University. Henry is single and lives in Chicago, where he spends his free time writing, reading, and enjoying music. He can be reached at hbnguyen@nwu.edu

SONAL SHAH

Sonal is a third-year medical student at Ross University. She currently resides in Southern California. She can be reached at sonal123@hotmail.com